hacking your hormone cycle

A WORKBOOK
for Finding Your Rhythm to Maximize Your
Energy, Productivity, and Happiness

SELENE WELLS

BLUESTONE BOOKS

Hacking Your Hormone Cycle.
Copyright © 2025 by Bluestone Books.
All rights reserved.

Any unauthorized duplication in whole or in part or dissemination of this edition by any means (including but not limited to photocopying, electronic devices, digital versions, and the internet) will be prosecuted to the fullest extent of the law.

Bluestone Books
www.bluestonebooks.co

Design by Joanna Price
Editorial by Jennifer Calvert
Special thanks to Kate Rispoli

ISBN: 978-1-965636-20-6 (paperback)

Printed in Canada
First Edition: 2025

10 9 8 7 6 5 4 3 2 1

IMPORTANT NOTE TO READERS: This book has been written and published for informational and educational purposes only. It is not intended to serve as medical advice or to be any form of medical treatment. You should always consult with your physician before altering or changing any aspect of your medical treatment. Do not stop or change any prescription medications without the guidance and advice of your physician. Any use of the information in this book is made on the reader's good judgment and is the reader's sole responsibility. This book is not intended to diagnose or treat any medical condition and is not a substitute for a physician.

Balance your hormones and take back your life!

We all know too well how fluctuating hormones impact our energy, moods, metabolism, and sleep. But did you know you can do something about it (besides trying to combat those fluctuations with caffeine, ibuprofen, chocolate, and sheer power of will)? You can work with your hormones all month long to make your life infinitely better. This holistic approach to wellness is called cycle syncing, and it takes just a few minor adjustments to your routine.

Although we tend to look at our daily habits as static, our bodies actually need us to be flexible. Different phases of the menstrual cycle require different levels of energy and different nutrients, all of which have different effects on our moods and mentality. By tailoring your habits to your hormonal fluctuations, you can finally get a good night's rest, be more productive at work and in your workouts, improve your relationships, enjoy great sex, and feel amazing—naturally!

You'll start by getting to know the four phases of your cycle: menstrual, follicular, ovulatory, and luteal. Each one comes with its own challenges but also imbues you with certain strengths. Knowing what those are means you can use them to your advantage. Increased testosterone during the ovulatory phase, for example, can give you the energy boost you need to hit the trails (or the sheets).

The magic happens when you track your cycle and begin to recognize its patterns. Maybe you tend to crave burgers on day one of your period—that could be your body telling you it needs more iron. Even your desire to curl up on the couch and watch TV during the menstrual phase is a hormonal cue. Your body needs rest to cleanse itself and prepare for the next phase of the cycle. Once you get a sense of your current habits, you can use the information you learn in the following pages to build on them.

So, start where you are with the daily tracking pages. Spend one full cycle just recording your habits, moods, sleep, food, and more in the context of your cycle. See if you can spot any patterns. Then begin to incorporate the cycle-specific advice for optimizing your wellness, and see how things shift. Once you've given the suggestions a chance to work, you can tweak your routines until you find what works best for you.

The Cycle Tracker at the back of the book lets you see your cycle and its effects at a glance. Do you always get annoying chin acne during your period? Flip back to your daily pages and see what you're eating in the last days of your luteal phase. You might want to swap that mac and cheese for some guacamole chicken salad. (Dairy can trigger breakouts.) Once you get a feel for your needs, the Activity Planner (just before the Cycle Tracker) lets you organize workouts, activities, and meals around your cycle. You can even start adding meals and movement to your daily pages to set yourself up for success. Before you know it, you'll have revolutionized your habits and feel better than you ever have.

IRREGULAR CYCLES & PERIMENOPAUSE

Although a menstrual cycle lasts twenty-eight days on average, every body is different. Anything between twenty-one and thirty-five days is completely normal. Once you hit perimenopause, though, you can experience irregular cycles with more or fewer bleeding days. That doesn't have to stop you from cycle syncing. In fact, the act of tracking your hormonal fluctuations can be especially beneficial during perimenopause. It helps you tailor your activity levels, sleep, and nutrition to your needs so you can find what feels good for you day by day.

The Menstrual Phase

DAYS 1–5 | WINTER | NEW MOON

Starting on the first full day of bleeding (not spotting), the menstrual phase lasts about five days on average. This is when your body sheds the thick uterine lining it has accumulated so it can begin a new cycle. Without a fertilized egg to cushion and support, your uterus no longer needs that tissue. But cleaning house is hard work. Fatigue is a common symptom, along with uterine cramps used to physically push out the unnecessary tissue lining. The drop in progesterone and estrogen can also cause headaches and migraines. That's why this phase is associated with winter—a time of rest and hibernation. On the plus side, much of the irritability, anxiety, and mood swings experienced in the days leading up to your period will quickly resolve once it arrives. And like the new moon, the menstrual phase offers a fresh start.

NUTRITION

As you shed your uterine lining, you're also shedding iron. This essential mineral is vital for healthy muscle function, brain development, and a strong immune system. So, during this phase, you'll want to supplement your diet with iron-rich foods. That could mean grabbing a burger on day one (typically the heaviest bleeding day), but red meat isn't the only good source of iron. Others include seafood, leafy green vegetables, nuts, legumes, beans, and dried fruits. Even an iron-enriched cereal can do the trick.

Salmon can be particularly helpful during the menstrual phase. It's not only a good source of iron, but its omega-3 fatty acids may also help mitigate cramping. These anti-inflammatory benefits can be found in other oily fish, walnuts, hemp seeds, flaxseeds, seaweed, eggs, and turmeric as well. Antioxidant-rich foods like berries, avocados, sweet potatoes, green tea, and—yes—dark chocolate can also be beneficial. As much as you might like to hunker down with some refined carbs and a glass of wine, avoiding sugary and fried foods and alcohol (which all increase inflammation) is going to help you feel good in your body right now.

> **TIP**
>
> Vitamin C can help your body absorb iron, whereas calcium can hinder iron absorption. So, serving your kale salad with citrus fruits and vegetables like broccoli, cauliflower, and bell peppers instead of calcium-rich foods like white beans can give you a boost.

EXERCISE

While your body works hard to start this new cycle, support it by taking it easy. Exercise is still helpful—it can energize you, clear your head, and reduce your pain. Instead of hitting the gym for a sweaty cycling class, though, choose a lower-impact workout like Pilates or yoga. The breathwork and stretching will feel great. You could also go for a walk. This isn't the time to push yourself. Listen to what your body needs, even if that means taking the day off.

SLEEP

In additional to your hormonal fluctuations and your bodily processes, you're literally losing blood during this phase. Rest is mandatory. Spend the evening curled up on the couch, take an afternoon nap if you need it, and sleep in if you can. Even an extra hour of sleep during this phase can make a huge difference in your energy levels.

SELF-CARE

Like winter, this is a good time for reflection and grounding. Listen to your body, set healthy boundaries, and step away from social media feeds (which can be especially exhausting during this phase). Sitting on the couch and binge-watching a favorite show, however, is encouraged, as is taking an Epsom-salts bath, which may help with any cramps. You could also go for a relaxing walk—breathing the fresh air and connecting with nature can help with the sense of overwhelm many people experience during this phase. This can be a great time for meditation and intention-setting. And if you're not up for cooking those nourishing foods you need, being in this phase is your excuse to order in.

RELATIONSHIPS

The same reflection and grounding that benefits you during this phase can benefit your interactions with friends and family. Be mindful to not let your physical discomfort manifest in your communication (i.e., don't take your cramps out on your partner). But this is a good time to work on asking for what you need (like alone time and a heating pad for those cramps).

Because estrogen is at its lowest point, sex is often not top of mind during the menstrual phase. But some people actually find themselves more aroused as the subsequent drop in progesterone makes way for both estrogen and testosterone to shine a bit. If that's you, you may need to use lubricant for the most enjoyable experience. Orgasms, with their endorphins and muscle contractions, are also a wonderful natural remedy for menstrual cramps. You might even find them more intense than at other times in your cycle.

WORK

As you may understand by now, the menstrual phase is not the best time for all-nighters, rush deadlines, and cooperative work. But it is a great time for deep thinking, planning, and prioritization. If you're able to carve out some alone time to quietly strategize, your work *and* your mood will benefit.

The Follicular Phase

DAYS 1–14 | SPRING | HALF MOON

Much like yourself, your body is always doing two things at once. The follicular phase starts at the same time as the menstrual phase (on the first day of your period). It typically lasts between ten and fourteen days and ends when ovulation begins. Like the waxing phase of the moon, this is a time for growth—literally and figuratively. Follicle-stimulating hormone (FSH) encourages follicles (the sacs that hold immature eggs) to develop in your ovaries, and a resulting boost in estrogen helps thicken your uterine lining. You'll feel your energy levels climbing and your creativity blooming, which is why this phase is the springtime of your cycle. Nourish it with estrogen-supporting foods and use that vibrant energy to your advantage in your daily movement, activities, and projects.

NUTRITION

In the first few days, which overlap with the menstrual phase, you'll want to continue seeking out iron-rich foods like red meat, spinach, and nuts. As your period ends, though, lean proteins and complex carbs (legumes and whole grains) will support your surging energy levels. They'll also help balance your blood sugar and repair your muscles as your desire to move naturally increases. Adding in healthy fats like avocados and cruciferous vegetables like broccoli and cauliflower can help level out your hormones for a smoother transition between phases.

If you plan to ramp up your exercise regimen during this phase, the anti-inflammatory foods that staved off menstrual pain will now help you stay active. Fatty fish, nuts and seeds, ginger and turmeric, berries, leafy green vegetables, and whole grains both fuel performance and aid muscle recovery. So does dark chocolate, by the way. And, of course, don't forget to hydrate!

> **TIP**
>
> If you're trying to get pregnant, this is the time to optimize your nutrition. Make sure your diet is rich in antioxidants, folate, omega-3 fatty acids, and lean proteins to support healthy follicle growth.

EXERCISE

As you start to come out of the fog of the menstrual phase and begin to feel more energized, you can switch to more high-impact workouts. Running, cycling, and cardio will all feel a little easier. If you really want to feel amazing, go outside and feel the sun on your face or try a fun and invigorating group fitness class. But, if you're not big on vigorous workouts, you can stick with low-impact exercises like walking, yoga, and Pilates. Any kind of movement will help balance your hormones and improve your mood—or, in the case of the follicular phase, sustain your already improved mood.

SLEEP

Sleep may be a little harder to come by later in the follicular phase thanks to rising progesterone levels. In other words, that buzz of energy you're feeling can seep into the evening hours. Moving more during the day (essentially tiring yourself out) can help. Make sure you're prioritizing rest, though, and not just staying awake longer. For one thing, sleep supports muscle recovery. For another, the luteal phase and its sleep-cycle interruptions are on the horizon.

SELF-CARE

You'll naturally feel more creative and curious during this phase, so focus on nurturing your mind. That could look like taking an art class or a hike in nature, journaling, making a vision board, or trying a new hobby. This is the time to dream big, make plans, and explore ideas. It's also a good time to make any uncomfortable self-care appointments (like waxing), because your pain tolerance rises with your estrogen levels. Just make sure to also nurture your body with plenty of rest, sunshine, and nourishment, just like you would a budding flower in spring.

RELATIONSHIPS

Once your desire to hibernate wears off, you'll begin to feel more social and look forward to plans with friends and family. Pair up for some of the self-care exercises that fuel you, like nature walks and new hobbies. You might also notice that you're more open to intimacy during the later days of the follicular phase. Because your body is setting the scene for ovulation and pregnancy, your libido begins to increase alongside your energy levels. Plus, your inhibitions are lowered and your confidence heightened (partly due to rising testosterone levels, and partly due to your skin clearing up). And increased lubrication makes everything more enjoyable. Of course, the days leading up to ovulation are your most fertile, so make sure you use protection if pregnancy isn't part of your plan.

WORK

Increases in creativity, curiosity, confidence, and motivation during the follicular phase can help you be your most productive at and outside of work. Use that boost in brainpower to tackle old problems and new projects, not to mention the plans you made during the menstrual phase. If there's a meeting or appointment you've been putting off, check it off your list during this phase. Each little victory adds to the feeling that you can take on the world. And because you'll be feeling more social, too, this is the perfect time to meet new people and network.

The Ovulatory Phase

DAYS 14–17 | SUMMER | FULL MOON

The ovulatory phase lasts just a few days, but everything in your cycle revolves around that short span. One of the follicles that started growing during the last phase has won the competition to become the best of them, bursting open and releasing a fully mature egg. That egg will travel into the fallopian tube and live for between twelve and twenty-four hours. (The fertilization window is longer than that, though—sperm can lie in wait for the egg for up to five days.) If the egg is not fertilized, your body will begin the process of shedding its lining. Whether or not you're trying to get pregnant, you can harness the summery energy and bright, full-moon optimism of the ovulatory phase to live your best life.

NUTRITION

Set yourself up for either a healthy conception or a slightly easier period with fewer premenstrual symptoms by balancing your rising estrogen with foods rich in fiber and antioxidants. Fatty fish, nuts, olive oil, edamame, oatmeal, vegetables, and fruits high in vitamin C work wonders. Cruciferous vegetables (like broccoli and cauliflower), in particular, release a compound that can help your liver break down estrogen. Steaming and sautéing rather than boiling or frying will help the food retain more of its nutrients, but eating fresh fruits and raw veggies is even better. And, of course, fueling your body with nourishing foods will also help you maximize the energy boost you get during the ovulatory phase.

If you're trying to conceive, add a B-complex vitamin to your daily regimen. It will help reduce the risk of early pregnancy complications and birth defects while supporting fetal brain development. You'll also want to start eating foods rich in iron and folic acid. (These happen to include fresh fruits and cruciferous vegetables.) No matter what, make sure you drink plenty of water and avoid salty and fatty foods, which can contribute to bloating during this phase.

TIP

One way to know when you're ovulating is to track your basal body temperature every day. It fluctuates slightly throughout your cycle and is at its highest point during ovulation, rising to between 97°F and 99°F from the typical 96°F to 98°F. For the most accurate readings, use a basal thermometer to take your temperature the minute you wake up in the morning—don't even get out of bed!

EXERCISE

Your energy began to ramp up during the follicular phase, and now it's summited the peak. You might get the urge to do the same. Embrace it. Go on an adventure. Get out and explore the world (or at least a local park). Climb a mountain, if that's your style. This is the time to push yourself physically. High-intensity interval workouts will feel less intense now than at other times during your cycle, as will cycling, hiking, circuits, cardio, and other demanding workouts. And they'll fuel your feel-good hormones.

SLEEP

That slight increase in body temperature, coupled with soaring energy levels, can make it harder to sleep during ovulation. Keep your room a little cooler, and make sure you wind down before bed (without your phone) for your best rest.

SELF-CARE

The ovulatory phase can make you feel invincible. Make the most of your superpowers by batch-cooking healthy meals, exercising, cleaning, and getting outside. With a little forward thinking, these days can set you up well for the rest of your cycle. This is a fertile time for ideas, too, so let yourself dream big. That's not to say ovulation doesn't have its downsides. You may experience *mittelschmerz*—German for "middle pain," it's the physical discomfort of feeling the egg's journey. It can last for a few minutes or up to two days. If you do have pain, rest and deep breaths can help. Your skin may also need a little pampering to combat acne, which can accompany ovulation's rise in testosterone.

RELATIONSHIPS

You're at your most open and social during the ovulatory phase, which makes it the perfect time to strike up conversations and forge new friendships. Your communication skills are also cresting, allowing you to more easily work out any disagreements. But the benefits to your relationships don't stop there. The increase in testosterone that gives you that lovely boost in energy and confidence will also rev up your sex drive. You'll notice more vaginal lubrication, feel more desirable, and enjoy even greater gratification. Physiologically, your body is creating an optimal environment for conception. Even if you're not trying to get pregnant, you can revel in this brief yet pleasurable experience.

WORK

Like your body, your brain is seeking stimulation during the ovulatory phase. Set up your most demanding tasks, meetings, and appointments during these days, when you're likely to be at your physical, mental, and emotional best. The luteal phase is coming quickly, bringing with it far less desire to tackle difficult projects. So do your future self a favor and check off anything on your to-do list that requires extra motivation or creativity. And make sure you don't say yes to anything now, when you're feeling on top of the world, that you'll have to do later, when you'd rather be under a blanket.

The Luteal Phase

DAYS 15-28 | AUTUMN | CRESCENT MOON

The luteal phase is the one that gets all the bad press, but there are plenty of ways to make the most of it through cycle syncing. During the first half of the phase, your body works to create an ideal environment for a fertilized egg. Estrogen and progesterone levels rise to prepare for implantation. Without a fertilized egg, those levels begin to wane like the crescent moon around day 22, ushering in the dreaded premenstrual syndrome (PMS). Tiredness and fatigue (yes, those are two different things), hunger and cravings, oily skin and acne, headaches, and even constipation are common as the uterus prepares to shed its lining. Thankfully, cycle syncing can help mitigate all of it. Greet the autumn of your cycle with slower movement, hearty nutrition, and an emphasis on your well-being.

NUTRITION

Wondering why you're so hungry? You can thank the luteal phase's hormonal cocktail. Focus on eating healthy fats that help you feel fuller, like avocados, and slow-digesting carbs, like sweet potatoes and beans. Of course, it's not just the hunger that gets you—it's also the cravings for salty and sweet. It's OK to give in to those hankerings sometimes, especially earlier on in the luteal phase. But you'll also want to incorporate healthier swaps to keep your blood sugar from spiking and spoiling your mood.

To allay other incoming PMS symptoms, support your body's progesterone production with vitamin B (particularly B_6) and increase your intake of magnesium, calcium, and soluble fiber. Beans, brown rice, berries, apples, and leafy greens pack the most nutritious punch, checking off more than one box each. These foods will help reduce inflammation, headaches, bloating, and constipation.

TIP

If you're prone to hormonal acne, be careful about which cravings you give in to—or, at least, how often you give in to them. Excess oil and sugar can trigger inflammation and breakouts.

EXERCISE

Think of the beginning of the luteal phase as the earlier months of autumn, and the end of the luteal phase as the later months. There's a big difference between a sunny September day and a chilly afternoon in early December. Start the phase with moderate workouts, ramping down from the more strenuous exercises of the late follicular phase. Strength training, less-intense cardio, and Pilates are all good choices. During the later days of the luteal phase, opt for gentler exercise, such as walking and yoga. Movement will help alleviate PMS symptoms, so try to squeeze in some form of it. But, first and foremost, listen to your body. If it's telling you to rest, you rest.

SLEEP

The luteal phase has the biggest impact on your sleep quality. Increased progesterone makes you want to curl up with a cozy blanket during the earlier days, but the later dip in estrogen can cause insomnia and a lack of deep, REM sleep. Working out during the day, not eating before bed, creating a calming sleep environment, and sticking to a consistent nighttime routine can help. And don't skimp on sleeping—your body needs more rest as you head into the menstrual phase.

SELF-CARE

Stress relief is going to be your top priority during the luteal phase. Meditation, deep-breathing exercises, journaling—do whatever helps you unclench your jaw. You'll also want to conserve your energy for important tasks, resting whenever possible. And, even though you may be feeling a little more stubborn than usual, accept help when you need it. Self-care is especially important if you're someone who suffers from premenstrual dysphoric disorder (PMDD), a severe form of PMS that can cause more upheaval during the late luteal phase.

RELATIONSHIPS

Although you're not feeling as social and outgoing, you'll find that the luteal phase does have its benefits to your relationships. You'll likely feel more focused and assertive during the later days of this phase. This may read as peevishness to some, but being able to cut to the chase and protect your time is essential when your energy levels (and patience) are lagging. Your sex drive will also be subdued and your lubrication lacking thanks to higher progesterone levels. That doesn't mean intimacy is off the table, just that you may need more foreplay and lubricant to enjoy it to the fullest. Most importantly, nurture your relationship with yourself during this phase.

WORK

This is the time to listen to your gut. Not only will you likely feel more introspective during the luteal phase, but you may also notice that your intuition is heightened. Use the resulting clarity to streamline processes and task lists, which will help with your ebbing energy levels. Your tolerance levels are also lower, so try to avoid group projects or interactions with coworkers who tend to push your buttons. Holing up in your office or cubicle and focusing on your priorities is the best thing you can do right now. You may not have the consistent vigor of the previous phases, but you can still align your work with your energy levels throughout the day. And don't give in to the nagging desire to give up. Like the luteal phase, it will pass.

JAN	FEB	MAR	APR	MAY	JUN	JUL	AUG	SEP	OCT	NOV	DEC
1	2	3	4	5	6	7	8	9	10	11	12	13	14	15	16
17	18	19	20	21	22	23	24	25	26	27	28	29	30	31

TRACK

Phase:

Mood:

Sleep:

Energy:

Symptoms:

Temperature:

PRIORITIZE

☐

☐

☐

NOURISH

B

L

D

+

MOVE

REPLENISH

HYDRATE

💧 💧 💧 💧 💧 💧 💧 💧

"With the new day comes new strength and new thoughts."

—ELEANOR ROOSEVELT

JAN	FEB	MAR	APR	MAY	JUN	JUL	AUG	SEP	OCT	NOV	DEC
1	2	3	4	5	6	7	8	9	10	11	12	13	14	15	16
17	18	19	20	21	22	23	24	25	26	27	28	29	30	31

TRACK

Phase:

Mood:

Sleep:

Energy:

Symptoms:

Temperature:

PRIORITIZE

☐

☐

☐

NOURISH

B

L

D

+

MOVE

REPLENISH

HYDRATE

💧 💧 💧 💧 💧 💧 💧 💧

TIP

The fatigue is real during the menstrual and luteal phases. Prioritizing rest (read: sleep) during those weeks is the best thing you can do for yourself.

JAN	FEB	MAR	APR	MAY	JUN	JUL	AUG	SEP	OCT	NOV	DEC
1	2	3	4	5	6	7	8	9	10	11	12	13	14	15	16
17	18	19	20	21	22	23	24	25	26	27	28	29	30	31

TRACK

Phase:

Mood:

Sleep:

Energy:

Symptoms:

Temperature:

PRIORITIZE

- [ ]
- [ ]
- [ ]

NOURISH

B

L

D

+

MOVE

REPLENISH

HYDRATE

💧 💧 💧 💧 💧 💧 💧 💧

"The secret of getting ahead is getting started."

—SALLY BERGER

JAN	FEB	MAR	APR	MAY	JUN	JUL	AUG	SEP	OCT	NOV	DEC
1	2	3	4	5	6	7	8	9	10	11	12	13	14	15	16
17	18	19	20	21	22	23	24	25	26	27	28	29	30	31

TRACK

Phase:

Mood:

Sleep:

Energy:

Symptoms:

Temperature:

PRIORITIZE

☐

☐

☐

NOURISH

B

L

D

+

MOVE

REPLENISH

HYDRATE

💧 💧 💧 💧 💧 💧 💧 💧

TIP

Don't let cycle syncing overwhelm you. Just set out to find what feels good, little by little.

JAN	FEB	MAR	APR	MAY	JUN	JUL	AUG	SEP	OCT	NOV	DEC
1	2	3	4	5	6	7	8	9	10	11	12	13	14	15	16
17	18	19	20	21	22	23	24	25	26	27	28	29	30	31

TRACK

Phase:

Mood:

Sleep:

Energy:

Symptoms:

Temperature:

PRIORITIZE

☐

☐

☐

NOURISH

B

L

D

+

MOVE

REPLENISH

HYDRATE

💧 💧 💧 💧 💧 💧 💧 💧

"I have chosen to no longer be apologetic for my femaleness and my femininity. And I want to be respected in all of my femaleness because I deserve to be."

—CHIMAMANDA NGOZI ADICHIE

JAN	FEB	MAR	APR	MAY	JUN	JUL	AUG	SEP	OCT	NOV	DEC
1	2	3	4	5	6	7	8	9	10	11	12	13	14	15	16
17	18	19	20	21	22	23	24	25	26	27	28	29	30	31	

TRACK

Phase:

Mood:

Sleep:

Energy:

Symptoms:

Temperature:

PRIORITIZE

☐

☐

☐

NOURISH

B

L

D

+

MOVE

REPLENISH

HYDRATE

💧 💧 💧 💧 💧 💧 💧 💧

TIP

You'll be at your most confident during your follicular phase, so use that time to schedule job interviews, first dates, or anything else that feels nerve-racking.

17

JAN	FEB	MAR	APR	MAY	JUN	JUL	AUG	SEP	OCT	NOV	DEC
1	2	3	4	5	6	7	8	9	10	11	12	13	14	15	16
17	18	19	20	21	22	23	24	25	26	27	28	29	30	31

TRACK

Phase:

Mood:

Sleep:

Energy:

Symptoms:

Temperature:

PRIORITIZE

- [ ]
- [ ]
- [ ]

NOURISH

B

L

D

+

MOVE

REPLENISH

HYDRATE

💧 💧 💧 💧 💧 💧 💧 💧

"It's our cycles that will get us where we want to be in life—we've got them, so let's use 'em!"

—MAISIE HILL

JAN	FEB	MAR	APR	MAY	JUN	JUL	AUG	SEP	OCT	NOV	DEC
1	2	3	4	5	6	7	8	9	10	11	12	13	14	15	16
17	18	19	20	21	22	23	24	25	26	27	28	29	30	31

TRACK

Phase:

Mood:

Sleep:

Energy:

Symptoms:

Temperature:

PRIORITIZE

☐

☐

☐

NOURISH

B

L

D

+

MOVE

REPLENISH

HYDRATE

💧 💧 💧 💧 💧 💧 💧 💧

TIP

Cycle syncing is about listening to your body, not just following guidelines. Make sure you adapt its advice to your own needs.

JAN	FEB	MAR	APR	MAY	JUN	JUL	AUG	SEP	OCT	NOV	DEC
1	2	3	4	5	6	7	8	9	10	11	12	13	14	15	16
17	18	19	20	21	22	23	24	25	26	27	28	29	30	31

TRACK

Phase:

Mood:

Sleep:

Energy:

Symptoms:

Temperature:

PRIORITIZE

- [ ]
- [ ]
- [ ]

NOURISH

B

L

D

+

MOVE

REPLENISH

HYDRATE

"Health is adding a level of intention to every area of your life."

—MIRANDA ANDERSON

JAN	FEB	MAR	APR	MAY	JUN	JUL	AUG	SEP	OCT	NOV	DEC
1	2	3	4	5	6	7	8	9	10	11	12	13	14	15	16
17	18	19	20	21	22	23	24	25	26	27	28	29	30	31

TRACK

Phase:

Mood:

Sleep:

Energy:

Symptoms:

Temperature:

PRIORITIZE

☐

☐

☐

NOURISH

B

L

D

+

MOVE

REPLENISH

HYDRATE

💧 💧 💧 💧 💧 💧 💧 💧

TIP

Try adding sesame seeds and sunflower seeds to your diet during the luteal phase to help balance increasing estrogen and waning progesterone.

JAN	FEB	MAR	APR	MAY	JUN	JUL	AUG	SEP	OCT	NOV	DEC
1	2	3	4	5	6	7	8	9	10	11	12	13	14	15	16
17	18	19	20	21	22	23	24	25	26	27	28	29	30	31

TRACK

Phase:

Mood:

Sleep:

Energy:

Symptoms:

Temperature:

PRIORITIZE

- [ ]
- [ ]
- [ ]

NOURISH

B

L

D

+

MOVE

REPLENISH

HYDRATE

💧 💧 💧 💧 💧 💧 💧 💧

"Knowledge is power, and the more knowledge you have of your body, the more power you have over your body."

—RACHEL McADAMS

22

JAN	FEB	MAR	APR	MAY	JUN	JUL	AUG	SEP	OCT	NOV	DEC
1	2	3	4	5	6	7	8	9	10	11	12	13	14	15	16
17	18	19	20	21	22	23	24	25	26	27	28	29	30	31

TRACK

Phase:

Mood:

Sleep:

Energy:

Symptoms:

Temperature:

PRIORITIZE

- [ ]
- [ ]
- [ ]

NOURISH

B

L

D

+

MOVE

REPLENISH

HYDRATE

TIP

Studies have found that periods are often longer, heavier, more painful, and more annoying during the winter months. Fight back by getting plenty of vitamin D.

JAN	FEB	MAR	APR	MAY	JUN	JUL	AUG	SEP	OCT	NOV	DEC
1	2	3	4	5	6	7	8	9	10	11	12	13	14	15	16
17	18	19	20	21	22	23	24	25	26	27	28	29	30	31

TRACK

Phase:

Mood:

Sleep:

Energy:

Symptoms:

Temperature:

PRIORITIZE

- [ ]
- [ ]
- [ ]

NOURISH

B

L

D

+

MOVE

REPLENISH

HYDRATE

💧 💧 💧 💧 💧 💧 💧 💧

"You must love and care for yourself, because that's when the best comes out."

—TINA TURNER

24

JAN	FEB	MAR	APR	MAY	JUN	JUL	AUG	SEP	OCT	NOV	DEC
1	2	3	4	5	6	7	8	9	10	11	12	13	14	15	16
17	18	19	20	21	22	23	24	25	26	27	28	29	30	31

TRACK

Phase:

Mood:

Sleep:

Energy:

Symptoms:

Temperature:

PRIORITIZE

☐
☐
☐

NOURISH

B

L

D

+

MOVE

REPLENISH

HYDRATE

💧 💧 💧 💧 💧 💧 💧

TIP

Eating cruciferous vegetables like broccoli, brussels sprouts, and cauliflower during the follicular phase will help balance rising estrogen levels and—bonus—boost your heart health.

25

JAN	FEB	MAR	APR	MAY	JUN	JUL	AUG	SEP	OCT	NOV	DEC
1	2	3	4	5	6	7	8	9	10	11	12	13	14	15	16
17	18	19	20	21	22	23	24	25	26	27	28	29	30	31

TRACK

Phase:

Mood:

Sleep:

Energy:

Symptoms:

Temperature:

PRIORITIZE

- [ ]
- [ ]
- [ ]

NOURISH

B

L

D

+

MOVE

REPLENISH

HYDRATE

○ ○ ○ ○ ○ ○ ○ ○

"When we're awake in our bodies and senses, the world comes alive. Wisdom, creativity, and love are discovered as we relax and awaken through our bodies."

—TARA BRACH

JAN	FEB	MAR	APR	MAY	JUN	JUL	AUG	SEP	OCT	NOV	DEC
1	2	3	4	5	6	7	8	9	10	11	12	13	14	15	16
17	18	19	20	21	22	23	24	25	26	27	28	29	30	31

TRACK

Phase:

Mood:

Sleep:

Energy:

Symptoms:

Temperature:

PRIORITIZE

- [ ]
- [ ]
- [ ]

NOURISH

B

L

D

+

MOVE

REPLENISH

HYDRATE

💧 💧 💧 💧 💧 💧 💧 💧

TIP

If you feel less inclined to have sex during ovulation (perhaps out of fear of conceiving), know that masturbation is also extra pleasurable during this phase.

JAN	FEB	MAR	APR	MAY	JUN	JUL	AUG	SEP	OCT	NOV	DEC
1	2	3	4	5	6	7	8	9	10	11	12	13	14	15	16
17	18	19	20	21	22	23	24	25	26	27	28	29	30	31

TRACK

Phase:

Mood:

Sleep:

Energy:

Symptoms:

Temperature:

PRIORITIZE

☐

☐

☐

NOURISH

B

L

D

+

MOVE

REPLENISH

HYDRATE

💧 💧 💧 💧 💧 💧 💧 💧

"To accept ourselves as we are means to value our imperfections as much as our perfections."

—SANDRA BIERIG

28

JAN	FEB	MAR	APR	MAY	JUN	JUL	AUG	SEP	OCT	NOV	DEC
1	2	3	4	5	6	7	8	9	10	11	12	13	14	15	16
17	18	19	20	21	22	23	24	25	26	27	28	29	30	31

TRACK

Phase:

Mood:

Sleep:

Energy:

Symptoms:

Temperature:

PRIORITIZE

☐

☐

☐

NOURISH

B

L

D

+

MOVE

REPLENISH

HYDRATE

TIP

Everyone's cycle is different! The average cycle lasts twenty-eight days, but yours might be as short as twenty-one or as long as thirty-five.

JAN	FEB	MAR	APR	MAY	JUN	JUL	AUG	SEP	OCT	NOV	DEC
1	2	3	4	5	6	7	8	9	10	11	12	13	14	15	16
17	18	19	20	21	22	23	24	25	26	27	28	29	30	31

TRACK

Phase:

Mood:

Sleep:

Energy:

Symptoms:

Temperature:

PRIORITIZE

- [ ]
- [ ]
- [ ]

NOURISH

B

L

D

+

MOVE

REPLENISH

HYDRATE

💧 💧 💧 💧 💧 💧 💧 💧

"Life is tough, my darling, but so are you."

—STEPHANIE BENNETT-HENRY

30

JAN	FEB	MAR	APR	MAY	JUN	JUL	AUG	SEP	OCT	NOV	DEC
1	2	3	4	5	6	7	8	9	10	11	12	13	14	15	16
17	18	19	20	21	22	23	24	25	26	27	28	29	30	31

TRACK

Phase:

Mood:

Sleep:

Energy:

Symptoms:

Temperature:

PRIORITIZE

☐

☐

☐

NOURISH

B

L

D

+

MOVE

REPLENISH

HYDRATE

💧 💧 💧 💧 💧 💧 💧

TIP

Counseling and cognitive behavioral therapy can help you feel like you have more agency over your body and can even help alleviate PMS.

JAN	FEB	MAR	APR	MAY	JUN	JUL	AUG	SEP	OCT	NOV	DEC
1	2	3	4	5	6	7	8	9	10	11	12	13	14	15	16
17	18	19	20	21	22	23	24	25	26	27	28	29	30	31

TRACK

Phase:

Mood:

Sleep:

Energy:

Symptoms:

Temperature:

PRIORITIZE

- [ ]
- [ ]
- [ ]

NOURISH

B

L

D

+

MOVE

REPLENISH

HYDRATE

💧 💧 💧 💧 💧 💧 💧 💧

"I am grateful to be a woman. I must have done something great in another life."

—MAYA ANGELOU

32

JAN	FEB	MAR	APR	MAY	JUN	JUL	AUG	SEP	OCT	NOV	DEC
1	2	3	4	5	6	7	8	9	10	11	12	13	14	15	16
17	18	19	20	21	22	23	24	25	26	27	28	29	30	31

TRACK

Phase:

Mood:

Sleep:

Energy:

Symptoms:

Temperature:

PRIORITIZE

☐

☐

☐

NOURISH

B

L

D

+

MOVE

REPLENISH

HYDRATE

💧 💧 💧 💧 💧 💧 💧 💧

TIP

Not only is there no harm in having sex while on your period, but the accompanying release of feel-good hormones dopamine and oxytocin can also boost your mood.

33

JAN	FEB	MAR	APR	MAY	JUN	JUL	AUG	SEP	OCT	NOV	DEC
1	2	3	4	5	6	7	8	9	10	11	12	13	14	15	16
17	18	19	20	21	22	23	24	25	26	27	28	29	30	31

TRACK

Phase:

Mood:

Sleep:

Energy:

Symptoms:

Temperature:

PRIORITIZE

- [ ]
- [ ]
- [ ]

NOURISH

B

L

D

+

MOVE

REPLENISH

HYDRATE

💧 💧 💧 💧 💧 💧 💧 💧

"Every day may not be good, but there is something good in every day."

—ALICE MORSE EARLE

JAN	FEB	MAR	APR	MAY	JUN	JUL	AUG	SEP	OCT	NOV	DEC
1	2	3	4	5	6	7	8	9	10	11	12	13	14	15	16
17	18	19	20	21	22	23	24	25	26	27	28	29	30	31

TRACK

Phase:

Mood:

Sleep:

Energy:

Symptoms:

Temperature:

PRIORITIZE

- [ ]
- [ ]
- [ ]

NOURISH

B

L

D

+

MOVE

REPLENISH

HYDRATE

TIP

Increased feelings of positivity during the follicular phase make this a great time to practice gratitude and nurture your mental health.

JAN	FEB	MAR	APR	MAY	JUN	JUL	AUG	SEP	OCT	NOV	DEC
1	2	3	4	5	6	7	8	9	10	11	12	13	14	15	16
17	18	19	20	21	22	23	24	25	26	27	28	29	30	31

TRACK

Phase:

Mood:

Sleep:

Energy:

Symptoms:

Temperature:

PRIORITIZE

☐

☐

☐

NOURISH

B

L

D

+

MOVE

REPLENISH

HYDRATE

💧 💧 💧 💧 💧 💧 💧 💧

"Your body is a temple, but only if you treat it as one."

—ASTRID ALAUDA

JAN	FEB	MAR	APR	MAY	JUN	JUL	AUG	SEP	OCT	NOV	DEC
1	2	3	4	5	6	7	8	9	10	11	12	13	14	15	16
17	18	19	20	21	22	23	24	25	26	27	28	29	30	31

TRACK

Phase:

Mood:

Sleep:

Energy:

Symptoms:

Temperature:

PRIORITIZE

- [ ]
- [ ]
- [ ]

NOURISH

B

L

D

+

MOVE

REPLENISH

HYDRATE

💧 💧 💧 💧 💧 💧 💧 💧

TIP

You can support your reproductive health by prioritizing foods that are rich in fiber (like brown rice and quinoa) and antioxidants (like berries and nuts) when you're ovulating.

37

JAN	FEB	MAR	APR	MAY	JUN	JUL	AUG	SEP	OCT	NOV	DEC
1	2	3	4	5	6	7	8	9	10	11	12	13	14	15	16
17	18	19	20	21	22	23	24	25	26	27	28	29	30	31

TRACK

Phase:

Mood:

Sleep:

Energy:

Symptoms:

Temperature:

PRIORITIZE

☐

☐

☐

NOURISH

B

L

D

+

MOVE

REPLENISH

HYDRATE

💧 💧 💧 💧 💧 💧 💧 💧

"Worry does not empty tomorrow of its sorrow. It empties today of its strength."

—CORRIE TEN BOOM

JAN	FEB	MAR	APR	MAY	JUN	JUL	AUG	SEP	OCT	NOV	DEC
1	2	3	4	5	6	7	8	9	10	11	12	13	14	15	16
17	18	19	20	21	22	23	24	25	26	27	28	29	30	31

TRACK

Phase:

Mood:

Sleep:

Energy:

Symptoms:

Temperature:

PRIORITIZE

☐

☐

☐

NOURISH

B

L

D

+

MOVE

REPLENISH

HYDRATE

💧 💧 💧 💧 💧 💧 💧

TIP

A short luteal phase (fewer than ten days) could indicate low progesterone. If you notice a pattern, bring your Cycle Tracker with you to talk to your healthcare provider.

39

JAN	FEB	MAR	APR	MAY	JUN	JUL	AUG	SEP	OCT	NOV	DEC
1	2	3	4	5	6	7	8	9	10	11	12	13	14	15	16
17	18	19	20	21	22	23	24	25	26	27	28	29	30	31

TRACK

Phase:

Mood:

Sleep:

Energy:

Symptoms:

Temperature:

PRIORITIZE

☐

☐

☐

NOURISH

B

L

D

+

MOVE

REPLENISH

HYDRATE

💧 💧 💧 💧 💧 💧 💧 💧

"Everybody is different, and every body is different."

—BEVERLY DIEHL

JAN	FEB	MAR	APR	MAY	JUN	JUL	AUG	SEP	OCT	NOV	DEC
1	2	3	4	5	6	7	8	9	10	11	12	13	14	15	16
17	18	19	20	21	22	23	24	25	26	27	28	29	30	31

TRACK

Phase:

Mood:

Sleep:

Energy:

Symptoms:

Temperature:

PRIORITIZE

☐

☐

☐

NOURISH

B

L

D

+

MOVE

REPLENISH

HYDRATE

💧 💧 💧 💧 💧 💧 💧

TIP

The best period product for you depends entirely on your comfort level, which is the priority during menstruation. No product is inherently better than another.

JAN	FEB	MAR	APR	MAY	JUN	JUL	AUG	SEP	OCT	NOV	DEC
1	2	3	4	5	6	7	8	9	10	11	12	13	14	15	16
17	18	19	20	21	22	23	24	25	26	27	28	29	30	31

TRACK

Phase:

Mood:

Sleep:

Energy:

Symptoms:

Temperature:

PRIORITIZE

☐

☐

☐

NOURISH

B

L

D

+

MOVE

REPLENISH

HYDRATE

💧 💧 💧 💧 💧 💧 💧 💧

"Every one of us needs to show how much we care for each other and, in the process, care for ourselves."

—PRINCESS DIANA

42

JAN	FEB	MAR	APR	MAY	JUN	JUL	AUG	SEP	OCT	NOV	DEC
1	2	3	4	5	6	7	8	9	10	11	12	13	14	15	16
17	18	19	20	21	22	23	24	25	26	27	28	29	30	31

TRACK

Phase:

Mood:

Sleep:

Energy:

Symptoms:

Temperature:

PRIORITIZE

- [ ]
- [ ]
- [ ]

NOURISH

B

L

D

+

MOVE

REPLENISH

HYDRATE

TIP

You'll be at your most social during the follicular phase, so use it to spend time out and about with friends and family.

43

JAN	FEB	MAR	APR	MAY	JUN	JUL	AUG	SEP	OCT	NOV	DEC
1	2	3	4	5	6	7	8	9	10	11	12	13	14	15	16
17	18	19	20	21	22	23	24	25	26	27	28	29	30	31

TRACK

Phase:

Mood:

Sleep:

Energy:

Symptoms:

Temperature:

PRIORITIZE

☐

☐

☐

NOURISH

B

L

D

+

MOVE

REPLENISH

HYDRATE

💧 💧 💧 💧 💧 💧 💧 💧

"Don't be intimidated by what you don't know. That can be your greatest strength and ensure that you do things differently from everyone else."

—SARA BLAKELY

44

JAN	FEB	MAR	APR	MAY	JUN	JUL	AUG	SEP	OCT	NOV	DEC
1	2	3	4	5	6	7	8	9	10	11	12	13	14	15	16
17	18	19	20	21	22	23	24	25	26	27	28	29	30	31

TRACK

Phase:

Mood:

Sleep:

Energy:

Symptoms:

Temperature:

PRIORITIZE

☐
☐
☐

NOURISH

B

L

D

+

MOVE

REPLENISH

HYDRATE

💧 💧 💧 💧 💧 💧 💧 💧

TIP

Progesterone decreases during perimenopause, causing effects similar to those of the luteal phase. Fill your diet with foods rich in vitamin B_6 (like avocados, bananas, and salmon) to support progesterone production.

45

JAN	FEB	MAR	APR	MAY	JUN	JUL	AUG	SEP	OCT	NOV	DEC
1	2	3	4	5	6	7	8	9	10	11	12	13	14	15	16
17	18	19	20	21	22	23	24	25	26	27	28	29	30	31

TRACK

Phase:

Mood:

Sleep:

Energy:

Symptoms:

Temperature:

PRIORITIZE

☐

☐

☐

NOURISH

B

L

D

+

MOVE

REPLENISH

HYDRATE

💧 💧 💧 💧 💧 💧 💧 💧

"A woman knows by intuition, or instinct, what is best for herself."

—MARILYN MONROE

JAN	FEB	MAR	APR	MAY	JUN	JUL	AUG	SEP	OCT	NOV	DEC
1	2	3	4	5	6	7	8	9	10	11	12	13	14	15	16
17	18	19	20	21	22	23	24	25	26	27	28	29	30	31

TRACK

Phase:

Mood:

Sleep:

Energy:

Symptoms:

Temperature:

PRIORITIZE

☐

☐

☐

NOURISH

B

L

D

+

MOVE

REPLENISH

HYDRATE

💧 💧 💧 💧 💧 💧 💧 💧

TIP

Use your luteal phase to reflect on how cycle syncing has been working for you, especially which habits have been making your life better.

47

JAN	FEB	MAR	APR	MAY	JUN	JUL	AUG	SEP	OCT	NOV	DEC
1	2	3	4	5	6	7	8	9	10	11	12	13	14	15	16
17	18	19	20	21	22	23	24	25	26	27	28	29	30	31

TRACK

Phase:

Mood:

Sleep:

Energy:

Symptoms:

Temperature:

PRIORITIZE

☐

☐

☐

NOURISH

B

L

D

+

MOVE

REPLENISH

HYDRATE

💧 💧 💧 💧 💧 💧 💧 💧

"Your skin is unique, so customize your routine accordingly."

—DR. ELLEN MARMUR

48

JAN	FEB	MAR	APR	MAY	JUN	JUL	AUG	SEP	OCT	NOV	DEC
1	2	3	4	5	6	7	8	9	10	11	12	13	14	15	16
17	18	19	20	21	22	23	24	25	26	27	28	29	30	31

TRACK

Phase:

Mood:

Sleep:

Energy:

Symptoms:

Temperature:

PRIORITIZE

☐

☐

☐

NOURISH

B

L

D

+

MOVE

REPLENISH

HYDRATE

TIP

Make sure your skin care routine features gentle products and a good moisturizer during your period to combat any dryness.

JAN	FEB	MAR	APR	MAY	JUN	JUL	AUG	SEP	OCT	NOV	DEC
1	2	3	4	5	6	7	8	9	10	11	12	13	14	15	16
17	18	19	20	21	22	23	24	25	26	27	28	29	30	31

TRACK

Phase:

Mood:

Sleep:

Energy:

Symptoms:

Temperature:

PRIORITIZE

☐

☐

☐

NOURISH

B

L

D

+

MOVE

REPLENISH

HYDRATE

💧 💧 💧 💧 💧 💧 💧 💧

"Everything is within your power, and your power is within you."

—JANICE TRACHTMAN

50

JAN	FEB	MAR	APR	MAY	JUN	JUL	AUG	SEP	OCT	NOV	DEC
1	2	3	4	5	6	7	8	9	10	11	12	13	14	15	16
17	18	19	20	21	22	23	24	25	26	27	28	29	30	31

TRACK

Phase:

Mood:

Sleep:

Energy:

Symptoms:

Temperature:

PRIORITIZE

☐

☐

☐

NOURISH

B

L

D

+

MOVE

REPLENISH

HYDRATE

💧 💧 💧 💧 💧 💧 💧 💧

TIP

The follicular phase makes your body more resilient, which makes this the best time for intense physical activity.

JAN	FEB	MAR	APR	MAY	JUN	JUL	AUG	SEP	OCT	NOV	DEC
1	2	3	4	5	6	7	8	9	10	11	12	13	14	15	16
17	18	19	20	21	22	23	24	25	26	27	28	29	30	31

TRACK

Phase:

Mood:

Sleep:

Energy:

Symptoms:

Temperature:

PRIORITIZE

- [ ]
- [ ]
- [ ]

NOURISH

B

L

D

+

MOVE

REPLENISH

HYDRATE

💧 💧 💧 💧 💧 💧 💧 💧

"Attention is vitality. It connects you with others. It makes you eager. Stay eager."

—SUSAN SONTAG

JAN	FEB	MAR	APR	MAY	JUN	JUL	AUG	SEP	OCT	NOV	DEC
1	2	3	4	5	6	7	8	9	10	11	12	13	14	15	16
17	18	19	20	21	22	23	24	25	26	27	28	29	30	31

TRACK

Phase:

Mood:

Sleep:

Energy:

Symptoms:

Temperature:

PRIORITIZE

☐

☐

☐

NOURISH

B

L

D

+

MOVE

REPLENISH

HYDRATE

💧 💧 💧 💧 💧 💧 💧 💧

TIP

Although a bit of discomfort during ovulation is normal, substantial pain is not. Listen to your body and talk to your healthcare provider if anything feels off.

JAN	FEB	MAR	APR	MAY	JUN	JUL	AUG	SEP	OCT	NOV	DEC
1	2	3	4	5	6	7	8	9	10	11	12	13	14	15	16
17	18	19	20	21	22	23	24	25	26	27	28	29	30	31

TRACK

Phase:

Mood:

Sleep:

Energy:

Symptoms:

Temperature:

PRIORITIZE

☐

☐

☐

NOURISH

B

L

D

+

MOVE

REPLENISH

HYDRATE

💧 💧 💧 💧 💧 💧 💧 💧

"You aren't doing 'nothing' when you choose to put your well-being first. In fact, this is the key to having everything."

—BRITTANY BURGUNDER

JAN	FEB	MAR	APR	MAY	JUN	JUL	AUG	SEP	OCT	NOV	DEC
1	2	3	4	5	6	7	8	9	10	11	12	13	14	15	16
17	18	19	20	21	22	23	24	25	26	27	28	29	30	31

TRACK

Phase:

Mood:

Sleep:

Energy:

Symptoms:

Temperature:

PRIORITIZE

☐
☐
☐

NOURISH

B

L

D

+

MOVE

REPLENISH

HYDRATE

💧 💧 💧 💧 💧 💧 💧 💧

TIP

Some days of your cycle will be harder on your mind, body, and emotions than others. Take rest when you need it.

JAN	FEB	MAR	APR	MAY	JUN	JUL	AUG	SEP	OCT	NOV	DEC
1	2	3	4	5	6	7	8	9	10	11	12	13	14	15	16
17	18	19	20	21	22	23	24	25	26	27	28	29	30	31

TRACK

Phase:

Mood:

Sleep:

Energy:

Symptoms:

Temperature:

PRIORITIZE

- [ ]
- [ ]
- [ ]

NOURISH

B

L

D

+

MOVE

REPLENISH

HYDRATE

💧 💧 💧 💧 💧 💧 💧 💧

"Small helpings. Sample a little bit of everything. These are the secrets of happiness and good health."

—JULIA CHILD

JAN	FEB	MAR	APR	MAY	JUN	JUL	AUG	SEP	OCT	NOV	DEC
1	2	3	4	5	6	7	8	9	10	11	12	13	14	15	16
17	18	19	20	21	22	23	24	25	26	27	28	29	30	31

TRACK

Phase:

Mood:

Sleep:

Energy:

Symptoms:

Temperature:

PRIORITIZE

☐
☐
☐

NOURISH

B

L

D

+

MOVE

REPLENISH

HYDRATE

💧 💧 💧 💧 💧 💧 💧

TIP

Eating five or six smaller meals throughout the day rather than three large meals can help minimize bloating and discomfort during the luteal phase.

JAN	FEB	MAR	APR	MAY	JUN	JUL	AUG	SEP	OCT	NOV	DEC
1	2	3	4	5	6	7	8	9	10	11	12	13	14	15	16
17	18	19	20	21	22	23	24	25	26	27	28	29	30	31

TRACK

Phase:

Mood:

Sleep:

Energy:

Symptoms:

Temperature:

PRIORITIZE

☐
☐
☐

NOURISH

B

L

D

+

MOVE

REPLENISH

HYDRATE

💧 💧 💧 💧 💧 💧 💧 💧

"One cannot think well, love well, sleep well, if one has not dined well."

—VIRGINIA WOOLF

JAN	FEB	MAR	APR	MAY	JUN	JUL	AUG	SEP	OCT	NOV	DEC
1	2	3	4	5	6	7	8	9	10	11	12	13	14	15	16
17	18	19	20	21	22	23	24	25	26	27	28	29	30	31

TRACK

Phase:

Mood:

Sleep:

Energy:

Symptoms:

Temperature:

PRIORITIZE

☐

☐

☐

NOURISH

B

L

D

+

MOVE

REPLENISH

HYDRATE

💧 💧 💧 💧 💧 💧 💧 💧

TIP

The best comfort foods to eat during your period are warm, nourishing meals, like soups and stews, that will boost your sense of well-being as well as your nutrients.

59

JAN	FEB	MAR	APR	MAY	JUN	JUL	AUG	SEP	OCT	NOV	DEC
1	2	3	4	5	6	7	8	9	10	11	12	13	14	15	16
17	18	19	20	21	22	23	24	25	26	27	28	29	30	31

TRACK

Phase:

Mood:

Sleep:

Energy:

Symptoms:

Temperature:

PRIORITIZE

- [ ]
- [ ]
- [ ]

NOURISH

B

L

D

+

MOVE

REPLENISH

HYDRATE

💧 💧 💧 💧 💧 💧 💧 💧

"Passion is energy. Feel the power that comes from focusing on what excites you."

—OPRAH WINFREY

JAN	FEB	MAR	APR	MAY	JUN	JUL	AUG	SEP	OCT	NOV	DEC
1	2	3	4	5	6	7	8	9	10	11	12	13	14	15	16
17	18	19	20	21	22	23	24	25	26	27	28	29	30	31

TRACK

Phase:

Mood:

Sleep:

Energy:

Symptoms:

Temperature:

PRIORITIZE

- [ ]
- [ ]
- [ ]

NOURISH

B

L

D

+

MOVE

REPLENISH

HYDRATE

TIP

Embrace feelings of motivation and curiosity during the follicular phase by trying a new activity. You may discover a new passion!

JAN	FEB	MAR	APR	MAY	JUN	JUL	AUG	SEP	OCT	NOV	DEC
1	2	3	4	5	6	7	8	9	10	11	12	13	14	15	16
17	18	19	20	21	22	23	24	25	26	27	28	29	30	31

TRACK

Phase:

Mood:

Sleep:

Energy:

Symptoms:

Temperature:

PRIORITIZE

- [ ]
- [ ]
- [ ]

NOURISH

B

L

D

+

MOVE

REPLENISH

HYDRATE

💧 💧 💧 💧 💧 💧 💧 💧

"Where there is love and inspiration, I don't think you can go wrong."

—ELLA FITZGERALD

JAN	FEB	MAR	APR	MAY	JUN	JUL	AUG	SEP	OCT	NOV	DEC
1	2	3	4	5	6	7	8	9	10	11	12	13	14	15	16
17	18	19	20	21	22	23	24	25	26	27	28	29	30	31

TRACK

Phase:

Mood:

Sleep:

Energy:

Symptoms:

Temperature:

PRIORITIZE

☐

☐

☐

NOURISH

B

L

D

+

MOVE

REPLENISH

HYDRATE

💧 💧 💧 💧 💧 💧 💧 💧

TIP

No one's pregnancy journey is the same. For some, conception happens quickly. But it's perfectly normal for it to take up to a year.

63

JAN	FEB	MAR	APR	MAY	JUN	JUL	AUG	SEP	OCT	NOV	DEC
1	2	3	4	5	6	7	8	9	10	11	12	13	14	15	16
17	18	19	20	21	22	23	24	25	26	27	28	29	30	31

TRACK

Phase:

Mood:

Sleep:

Energy:

Symptoms:

Temperature:

PRIORITIZE

- [ ]
- [ ]
- [ ]

NOURISH

B

L

D

+

MOVE

REPLENISH

HYDRATE

💧 💧 💧 💧 💧 💧 💧

"Your body is your best guide. It constantly tells you, in the form of pain or sensations, what's working for you and what's not."

—HINA HASHMI

JAN	FEB	MAR	APR	MAY	JUN	JUL	AUG	SEP	OCT	NOV	DEC
1	2	3	4	5	6	7	8	9	10	11	12	13	14	15	16
17	18	19	20	21	22	23	24	25	26	27	28	29	30	31	

TRACK

Phase:

Mood:

Sleep:

Energy:

Symptoms:

Temperature:

PRIORITIZE

- [ ]
- [ ]
- [ ]

NOURISH

B

L

D

+

MOVE

REPLENISH

HYDRATE

TIP

Think of your menstrual cycle as a vital sign, like blood pressure or oxygen saturation. It can give you insight into how your whole body is functioning.

JAN	FEB	MAR	APR	MAY	JUN	JUL	AUG	SEP	OCT	NOV	DEC
1	2	3	4	5	6	7	8	9	10	11	12	13	14	15	16
17	18	19	20	21	22	23	24	25	26	27	28	29	30	31

TRACK

Phase:

Mood:

Sleep:

Energy:

Symptoms:

Temperature:

PRIORITIZE

- [ ]
- [ ]
- [ ]

NOURISH

B

L

D

+

MOVE

REPLENISH

HYDRATE

"Write down the things that are on your mind. The simple act of listing your thoughts can have a cathartic and healing effect."

—JULIA LAFLIN

JAN	FEB	MAR	APR	MAY	JUN	JUL	AUG	SEP	OCT	NOV	DEC
1	2	3	4	5	6	7	8	9	10	11	12	13	14	15	16
17	18	19	20	21	22	23	24	25	26	27	28	29	30	31

TRACK

Phase:

Mood:

Sleep:

Energy:

Symptoms:

Temperature:

PRIORITIZE

- [ ]
- [ ]
- [ ]

NOURISH

B

L

D

+

MOVE

REPLENISH

HYDRATE

💧 💧 💧 💧 💧 💧 💧 💧

TIP

Keeping a journal during the luteal phase can help you feel less stressed and, therefore, be less reactive during this phase.

JAN	FEB	MAR	APR	MAY	JUN	JUL	AUG	SEP	OCT	NOV	DEC
1	2	3	4	5	6	7	8	9	10	11	12	13	14	15	16
17	18	19	20	21	22	23	24	25	26	27	28	29	30	31

TRACK

Phase:

Mood:

Sleep:

Energy:

Symptoms:

Temperature:

PRIORITIZE

- [ ]
- [ ]
- [ ]

NOURISH

B

L

D

+

MOVE

REPLENISH

HYDRATE

💧💧💧💧💧💧💧💧

"If my world were to cave in tomorrow, I would look back on all the pleasures, excitements, and worthwhilenesses I have been lucky enough to have had."

—AUDREY HEPBURN

JAN	FEB	MAR	APR	MAY	JUN	JUL	AUG	SEP	OCT	NOV	DEC
1	2	3	4	5	6	7	8	9	10	11	12	13	14	15	16
17	18	19	20	21	22	23	24	25	26	27	28	29	30	31

TRACK

Phase:

Mood:

Sleep:

Energy:

Symptoms:

Temperature:

PRIORITIZE

☐

☐

☐

NOURISH

B

L

D

+

MOVE

REPLENISH

HYDRATE

💧 💧 💧 💧 💧 💧 💧 💧

TIP

Whether you're alone or with a partner, endorphins released during orgasm can make menstrual cramps feel better.

JAN	FEB	MAR	APR	MAY	JUN	JUL	AUG	SEP	OCT	NOV	DEC
1	2	3	4	5	6	7	8	9	10	11	12	13	14	15	16
17	18	19	20	21	22	23	24	25	26	27	28	29	30	31

TRACK

Phase:

Mood:

Sleep:

Energy:

Symptoms:

Temperature:

PRIORITIZE

- [ ]
- [ ]
- [ ]

NOURISH

B

L

D

+

MOVE

REPLENISH

HYDRATE

💧 💧 💧 💧 💧 💧 💧 💧

"Your body is the direct result of what you eat as well as what you don't eat."

—GLORIA SWANSON

JAN	FEB	MAR	APR	MAY	JUN	JUL	AUG	SEP	OCT	NOV	DEC
1	2	3	4	5	6	7	8	9	10	11	12	13	14	15	16
17	18	19	20	21	22	23	24	25	26	27	28	29	30	31

TRACK

Phase:

Mood:

Sleep:

Energy:

Symptoms:

Temperature:

PRIORITIZE

- [ ]
- [ ]
- [ ]

NOURISH

B

L

D

+

MOVE

REPLENISH

HYDRATE

◇ ◇ ◇ ◇ ◇ ◇ ◇ ◇

TIP

If you gave in to cravings of salty or sweet during the menstrual phase, make up for it with nourishing foods that feed your rising energy levels during the follicular phase.

JAN	FEB	MAR	APR	MAY	JUN	JUL	AUG	SEP	OCT	NOV	DEC
1	2	3	4	5	6	7	8	9	10	11	12	13	14	15	16
17	18	19	20	21	22	23	24	25	26	27	28	29	30	31

TRACK

Phase:

Mood:

Sleep:

Energy:

Symptoms:

Temperature:

PRIORITIZE

☐

☐

☐

NOURISH

B

L

D

+

MOVE

REPLENISH

HYDRATE

💧 💧 💧 💧 💧 💧 💧 💧

"You are the most constant thing in your own life. Befriend yourself first. Invest in yourself first. Become yourself first. The rest will come together in time."

—BRIANNA WIEST

JAN	FEB	MAR	APR	MAY	JUN	JUL	AUG	SEP	OCT	NOV	DEC
1	2	3	4	5	6	7	8	9	10	11	12	13	14	15	16
17	18	19	20	21	22	23	24	25	26	27	28	29	30	31	

TRACK

Phase:

Mood:

Sleep:

Energy:

Symptoms:

Temperature:

MOVE

PRIORITIZE

☐

☐

☐

REPLENISH

NOURISH

B

L

D

+

HYDRATE

💧 💧 💧 💧 💧 💧 💧 💧

TIP

Whether you're trying to get pregnant, minimize period pain, maximize your productivity, or just feel more connected to your body, consistent tracking is key.

JAN	FEB	MAR	APR	MAY	JUN	JUL	AUG	SEP	OCT	NOV	DEC
1	2	3	4	5	6	7	8	9	10	11	12	13	14	15	16
17	18	19	20	21	22	23	24	25	26	27	28	29	30	31

TRACK

Phase:

Mood:

Sleep:

Energy:

Symptoms:

Temperature:

PRIORITIZE

☐

☐

☐

NOURISH

B

L

D

+

MOVE

REPLENISH

HYDRATE

💧 💧 💧 💧 💧 💧 💧 💧

"We are indeed much more than what we eat, but what we eat can nevertheless help us to be much more than what we are."

—ADELLE DAVIS

JAN	FEB	MAR	APR	MAY	JUN	JUL	AUG	SEP	OCT	NOV	DEC
1	2	3	4	5	6	7	8	9	10	11	12	13	14	15	16
17	18	19	20	21	22	23	24	25	26	27	28	29	30	31

TRACK

Phase:

Mood:

Sleep:

Energy:

Symptoms:

Temperature:

PRIORITIZE

☐

☐

☐

NOURISH

B

L

D

+

MOVE

REPLENISH

HYDRATE

💧 💧 💧 💧 💧 💧 💧

TIP

Your metabolism revs up during your luteal phase, so you'll need to eat more calories to stabilize your blood sugar (and your mood).

JAN	FEB	MAR	APR	MAY	JUN	JUL	AUG	SEP	OCT	NOV	DEC
1	2	3	4	5	6	7	8	9	10	11	12	13	14	15	16
17	18	19	20	21	22	23	24	25	26	27	28	29	30	31

TRACK

Phase:

Mood:

Sleep:

Energy:

Symptoms:

Temperature:

PRIORITIZE

- [ ]
- [ ]
- [ ]

NOURISH

B

L

D

+

MOVE

REPLENISH

HYDRATE

💧 💧 💧 💧 💧 💧 💧 💧

"If you want to meet your goals, you have to make it about you. You have to make it work for you and you alone."

—JENNIFER HUDSON

JAN	FEB	MAR	APR	MAY	JUN	JUL	AUG	SEP	OCT	NOV	DEC
1	2	3	4	5	6	7	8	9	10	11	12	13	14	15	16
17	18	19	20	21	22	23	24	25	26	27	28	29	30	31

TRACK

Phase:

Mood:

Sleep:

Energy:

Symptoms:

Temperature:

PRIORITIZE

☐

☐

☐

NOURISH

B

L

D

+

MOVE

REPLENISH

HYDRATE

💧 💧 💧 💧 💧 💧 💧 💧

TIP

Don't worry about keeping up with others during your menstrual phase—focus on listening to your own body.

77

JAN	FEB	MAR	APR	MAY	JUN	JUL	AUG	SEP	OCT	NOV	DEC
1	2	3	4	5	6	7	8	9	10	11	12	13	14	15	16
17	18	19	20	21	22	23	24	25	26	27	28	29	30	31

TRACK

Phase:

Mood:

Sleep:

Energy:

Symptoms:

Temperature:

PRIORITIZE

- [ ]
- [ ]
- [ ]

NOURISH

B

L

D

+

MOVE

REPLENISH

HYDRATE

"Nourishing yourself in a way that helps you blossom in the direction you want to go is attainable, and you are worth the effort."

—DEBORAH DAY

78

JAN	FEB	MAR	APR	MAY	JUN	JUL	AUG	SEP	OCT	NOV	DEC
1	2	3	4	5	6	7	8	9	10	11	12	13	14	15	16
17	18	19	20	21	22	23	24	25	26	27	28	29	30	31	

TRACK

Phase:

Mood:

Sleep:

Energy:

Symptoms:

Temperature:

PRIORITIZE

☐

☐

☐

NOURISH

B

L

D

+

MOVE

REPLENISH

HYDRATE

TIP

Take advantage of the energy boost you get from the follicular phase and try a new high-impact workout or exercise class.

79

JAN	FEB	MAR	APR	MAY	JUN	JUL	AUG	SEP	OCT	NOV	DEC
1	2	3	4	5	6	7	8	9	10	11	12	13	14	15	16
17	18	19	20	21	22	23	24	25	26	27	28	29	30	31

TRACK

Phase:

Mood:

Sleep:

Energy:

Symptoms:

Temperature:

PRIORITIZE

☐

☐

☐

NOURISH

B

L

D

+

MOVE

REPLENISH

HYDRATE

💧 💧 💧 💧 💧 💧 💧 💧

"We think the vagina is on the outside. I say grab a mirror and play along. Get in there. Learn about it."

—CAMERON DIAZ

80

JAN	FEB	MAR	APR	MAY	JUN	JUL	AUG	SEP	OCT	NOV	DEC
1	2	3	4	5	6	7	8	9	10	11	12	13	14	15	16
17	18	19	20	21	22	23	24	25	26	27	28	29	30	31

TRACK

Phase:

Mood:

Sleep:

Energy:

Symptoms:

Temperature:

PRIORITIZE

- [ ]
- [ ]
- [ ]

NOURISH

B

L

D

+

MOVE

REPLENISH

HYDRATE

TIP

One way to know whether you're ovulating: your cervical mucus will be thicker and more slippery (to help sperm successfully make it to an egg).

JAN	FEB	MAR	APR	MAY	JUN	JUL	AUG	SEP	OCT	NOV	DEC
1	2	3	4	5	6	7	8	9	10	11	12	13	14	15	16
17	18	19	20	21	22	23	24	25	26	27	28	29	30	31

TRACK

Phase:

Mood:

Sleep:

Energy:

Symptoms:

Temperature:

PRIORITIZE

- [ ]
- [ ]
- [ ]

NOURISH

B

L

D

+

MOVE

REPLENISH

HYDRATE

💧 💧 💧 💧 💧 💧 💧 💧

"We cannot change what we are not aware of, and once we are aware, we cannot help but change."

—SHERYL SANDBERG

82

JAN	FEB	MAR	APR	MAY	JUN	JUL	AUG	SEP	OCT	NOV	DEC
1	2	3	4	5	6	7	8	9	10	11	12	13	14	15	16
17	18	19	20	21	22	23	24	25	26	27	28	29	30	31

TRACK

Phase:

Mood:

Sleep:

Energy:

Symptoms:

Temperature:

PRIORITIZE

- [ ]
- [ ]
- [ ]

NOURISH

B

L

D

+

MOVE

REPLENISH

HYDRATE

💧 💧 💧 💧 💧 💧 💧 💧

TIP

You can still benefit from cycle syncing if you use a hormonal contraceptive that suppresses ovulation. Just pay attention to your body's needs and adjust your routine accordingly.

JAN	FEB	MAR	APR	MAY	JUN	JUL	AUG	SEP	OCT	NOV	DEC
1	2	3	4	5	6	7	8	9	10	11	12	13	14	15	16
17	18	19	20	21	22	23	24	25	26	27	28	29	30	31

TRACK

Phase:

Mood:

Sleep:

Energy:

Symptoms:

Temperature:

PRIORITIZE

☐

☐

☐

NOURISH

B

L

D

+

MOVE

REPLENISH

HYDRATE

💧 💧 💧 💧 💧 💧 💧 💧

"There must be quite a few things a hot bath won't cure, but I don't know many of them."

—SYLVIA PLATH

JAN	FEB	MAR	APR	MAY	JUN	JUL	AUG	SEP	OCT	NOV	DEC
1	2	3	4	5	6	7	8	9	10	11	12	13	14	15	16
17	18	19	20	21	22	23	24	25	26	27	28	29	30	31

TRACK

Phase:

Mood:

Sleep:

Energy:

Symptoms:

Temperature:

PRIORITIZE

☐

☐

☐

NOURISH

B

L

D

+

MOVE

REPLENISH

HYDRATE

TIP

To mitigate the luteal phase's impact on your sleep, try winding down before bed with a good book, some calming music, and a warm bath. (And avoid screens!)

JAN	FEB	MAR	APR	MAY	JUN	JUL	AUG	SEP	OCT	NOV	DEC
1	2	3	4	5	6	7	8	9	10	11	12	13	14	15	16
17	18	19	20	21	22	23	24	25	26	27	28	29	30	31

TRACK

Phase:

Mood:

Sleep:

Energy:

Symptoms:

Temperature:

PRIORITIZE

☐

☐

☐

NOURISH

B

L

D

+

MOVE

REPLENISH

HYDRATE

💧 💧 💧 💧 💧 💧 💧 💧

"Real rest feels like every cell is thanking you for taking care of you."

—JENNIFER WILLIAMSON

JAN	FEB	MAR	APR	MAY	JUN	JUL	AUG	SEP	OCT	NOV	DEC
1	2	3	4	5	6	7	8	9	10	11	12	13	14	15	16
17	18	19	20	21	22	23	24	25	26	27	28	29	30	31

TRACK

Phase:

Mood:

Sleep:

Energy:

Symptoms:

Temperature:

PRIORITIZE

- [ ]
- [ ]
- [ ]

NOURISH

B

L

D

+

MOVE

REPLENISH

HYDRATE

💧 💧 💧 💧 💧 💧 💧

TIP

If you have trouble sleeping while on your period, try lowering the room temperature and wearing light clothing to regulate your body temperature.

JAN	FEB	MAR	APR	MAY	JUN	JUL	AUG	SEP	OCT	NOV	DEC
1	2	3	4	5	6	7	8	9	10	11	12	13	14	15	16
17	18	19	20	21	22	23	24	25	26	27	28	29	30	31

TRACK

Phase:

Mood:

Sleep:

Energy:

Symptoms:

Temperature:

PRIORITIZE

- [ ]
- [ ]
- [ ]

NOURISH

B

L

D

+

MOVE

REPLENISH

HYDRATE

💧 💧 💧 💧 💧 💧 💧 💧

"I can do and be whatever I want to be because I proved to myself and everyone around me how strong I am."

—AMBER DENAE WRIGHT

JAN	FEB	MAR	APR	MAY	JUN	JUL	AUG	SEP	OCT	NOV	DEC
1	2	3	4	5	6	7	8	9	10	11	12	13	14	15	16
17	18	19	20	21	22	23	24	25	26	27	28	29	30	31

TRACK

Phase:

Mood:

Sleep:

Energy:

Symptoms:

Temperature:

PRIORITIZE

☐

☐

☐

NOURISH

B

L

D

+

MOVE

REPLENISH

HYDRATE

💧 💧 💧 💧 💧 💧 💧

TIP

Your pain tolerance will be at its highest toward the end of the follicular phase, so it's a good time to schedule potentially painful activities, like dental work (or getting a new tattoo).

89

JAN	FEB	MAR	APR	MAY	JUN	JUL	AUG	SEP	OCT	NOV	DEC
1	2	3	4	5	6	7	8	9	10	11	12	13	14	15	16
17	18	19	20	21	22	23	24	25	26	27	28	29	30	31

TRACK

Phase:

Mood:

Sleep:

Energy:

Symptoms:

Temperature:

PRIORITIZE

☐

☐

☐

NOURISH

B

L

D

+

MOVE

REPLENISH

HYDRATE

💧 💧 💧 💧 💧 💧 💧 💧

"Making the decision to have a child—it's momentous. It is to decide forever to have your heart go walking around outside your body."

—ELIZABETH STONE

JAN	FEB	MAR	APR	MAY	JUN	JUL	AUG	SEP	OCT	NOV	DEC
1	2	3	4	5	6	7	8	9	10	11	12	13	14	15	16
17	18	19	20	21	22	23	24	25	26	27	28	29	30	31

TRACK

Phase:

Mood:

Sleep:

Energy:

Symptoms:

Temperature:

PRIORITIZE

- [ ]
- [ ]
- [ ]

NOURISH

B

L

D

+

MOVE

REPLENISH

HYDRATE

💧 💧 💧 💧 💧 💧 💧 💧

TIP

Irregular cycles don't necessarily make it harder to conceive, but fertility experts can help things along with medications that induce ovulation if needed.

JAN	FEB	MAR	APR	MAY	JUN	JUL	AUG	SEP	OCT	NOV	DEC
1	2	3	4	5	6	7	8	9	10	11	12	13	14	15	16
17	18	19	20	21	22	23	24	25	26	27	28	29	30	31

TRACK

Phase:

Mood:

Sleep:

Energy:

Symptoms:

Temperature:

PRIORITIZE

- [ ]
- [ ]
- [ ]

NOURISH

B

L

D

+

MOVE

REPLENISH

HYDRATE

💧 💧 💧 💧 💧 💧 💧 💧

"Your skin is a lifelong investment; treat it with care."

—DR. SHEREENE IDRISS

JAN	FEB	MAR	APR	MAY	JUN	JUL	AUG	SEP	OCT	NOV	DEC
1	2	3	4	5	6	7	8	9	10	11	12
13	14	15	16	17	18	19	20	21	22	23	24
25	26	27	28	29	30	31					

TRACK

Phase:

Mood:

Sleep:

Energy:

Symptoms:

Temperature:

PRIORITIZE

- [ ]
- [ ]
- [ ]

NOURISH

B

L

D

+

MOVE

REPLENISH

HYDRATE

💧 💧 💧 💧 💧 💧 💧 💧

TIP

Although your skin will feel oilier during the luteal phase, don't skip your moisturizer. A lightweight product will help protect your skin's moisture barrier and prevent oil overproduction.

JAN	FEB	MAR	APR	MAY	JUN	JUL	AUG	SEP	OCT	NOV	DEC
1	2	3	4	5	6	7	8	9	10	11	12	13	14	15	16
17	18	19	20	21	22	23	24	25	26	27	28	29	30	31

TRACK

Phase:

Mood:

Sleep:

Energy:

Symptoms:

Temperature:

PRIORITIZE

- [ ]
- [ ]
- [ ]

NOURISH

B

L

D

+

MOVE

REPLENISH

HYDRATE

💧 💧 💧 💧 💧 💧 💧 💧

"Love yourself enough to set boundaries. Your time and energy are precious. You get to choose how you use it."

—ANNA TAYLOR

JAN	FEB	MAR	APR	MAY	JUN	JUL	AUG	SEP	OCT	NOV	DEC
1	2	3	4	5	6	7	8	9	10	11	12	13	14	15	16
17	18	19	20	21	22	23	24	25	26	27	28	29	30	31

TRACK

Phase:

Mood:

Sleep:

Energy:

Symptoms:

Temperature:

PRIORITIZE

- [ ]
- [ ]
- [ ]

NOURISH

B

L

D

+

MOVE

REPLENISH

HYDRATE

TIP

During the menstrual phase, focus on self-care to help with increased emotional vulnerability: avoid stressors, set boundaries, and prioritize rest when you can.

JAN	FEB	MAR	APR	MAY	JUN	JUL	AUG	SEP	OCT	NOV	DEC
1	2	3	4	5	6	7	8	9	10	11	12	13	14	15	16
17	18	19	20	21	22	23	24	25	26	27	28	29	30	31

TRACK

Phase:

Mood:

Sleep:

Energy:

Symptoms:

Temperature:

PRIORITIZE

- [ ]
- [ ]
- [ ]

NOURISH

B

L

D

+

MOVE

REPLENISH

HYDRATE

💧 💧 💧 💧 💧 💧 💧 💧

"Menopause is an opportunity to gracefully let go of what no longer serves you and welcome in new possibilities."

—DR. CHRISTIANE NORTHRUP

96

JAN	FEB	MAR	APR	MAY	JUN	JUL	AUG	SEP	OCT	NOV	DEC
1	2	3	4	5	6	7	8	9	10	11	12	13	14	15	16
17	18	19	20	21	22	23	24	25	26	27	28	29	30	31

TRACK

Phase:

Mood:

Sleep:

Energy:

Symptoms:

Temperature:

MOVE

REPLENISH

PRIORITIZE

- [ ]
- [ ]
- [ ]

NOURISH

B

L

D

+

HYDRATE

TIP

A shorter follicular phase can indicate that you're in or inching closer to perimenopause. Look for other symptoms, such as night sweats or heart palpitations.

97

JAN	FEB	MAR	APR	MAY	JUN	JUL	AUG	SEP	OCT	NOV	DEC
1	2	3	4	5	6	7	8	9	10	11	12	13	14	15	16
17	18	19	20	21	22	23	24	25	26	27	28	29	30	31

TRACK

Phase:

Mood:

Sleep:

Energy:

Symptoms:

Temperature:

PRIORITIZE

- [ ]
- [ ]
- [ ]

NOURISH

B

L

D

+

MOVE

REPLENISH

HYDRATE

💧 💧 💧 💧 💧 💧 💧 💧

"You must love yourself internally to glow externally."

—HANNAH BRONFMAN

JAN	FEB	MAR	APR	MAY	JUN	JUL	AUG	SEP	OCT	NOV	DEC
1	2	3	4	5	6	7	8	9	10	11	12	13	14	15	16
17	18	19	20	21	22	23	24	25	26	27	28	29	30	31

TRACK

Phase:

Mood:

Sleep:

Energy:

Symptoms:

Temperature:

PRIORITIZE

- [ ]
- [ ]
- [ ]

NOURISH

B

L

D

+

MOVE

REPLENISH

HYDRATE

TIP

When cycle syncing, make sure you're looking at the whole picture. Note any changes you experience in your mood, mindset, energy, sleep, and skin.

JAN	FEB	MAR	APR	MAY	JUN	JUL	AUG	SEP	OCT	NOV	DEC
1	2	3	4	5	6	7	8	9	10	11	12	13	14	15	16
17	18	19	20	21	22	23	24	25	26	27	28	29	30	31

TRACK

Phase:

Mood:

Sleep:

Energy:

Symptoms:

Temperature:

PRIORITIZE

- [ ]
- [ ]
- [ ]

NOURISH

B

L

D

+

MOVE

REPLENISH

HYDRATE

💧 💧 💧 💧 💧 💧 💧 💧

"You are a VIP, a very important person. So take care with self-care. If not you, who? If not now, when?"

—TONI HAWKINS

JAN	FEB	MAR	APR	MAY	JUN	JUL	AUG	SEP	OCT	NOV	DEC
1	2	3	4	5	6	7	8	9	10	11	12	13	14	15	16
17	18	19	20	21	22	23	24	25	26	27	28	29	30	31

TRACK

Phase:

Mood:

Sleep:

Energy:

Symptoms:

Temperature:

PRIORITIZE

- [ ]
- [ ]
- [ ]

NOURISH

B

L

D

+

MOVE

REPLENISH

HYDRATE

TIP

Hydration is key during the luteal phase: strive to drink at least eight glasses of water a day to minimize bloating and aid digestion.

JAN	FEB	MAR	APR	MAY	JUN	JUL	AUG	SEP	OCT	NOV	DEC
1	2	3	4	5	6	7	8	9	10	11	12	13	14	15	16
17	18	19	20	21	22	23	24	25	26	27	28	29	30	31

TRACK

Phase:

Mood:

Sleep:

Energy:

Symptoms:

Temperature:

PRIORITIZE

- [ ]
- [ ]
- [ ]

NOURISH

B

L

D

+

MOVE

REPLENISH

HYDRATE

💧 💧 💧 💧 💧 💧 💧 💧

"Let go of who you think you're supposed to be and embrace who you are."

—BRENÉ BROWN

JAN	FEB	MAR	APR	MAY	JUN	JUL	AUG	SEP	OCT	NOV	DEC
1	2	3	4	5	6	7	8	9	10	11	12	13	14	15	16
17	18	19	20	21	22	23	24	25	26	27	28	29	30	31

TRACK

Phase:

Mood:

Sleep:

Energy:

Symptoms:

Temperature:

PRIORITIZE

- [ ]
- [ ]
- [ ]

NOURISH

B

L

D

+

MOVE

REPLENISH

HYDRATE

TIP

Remember that the vagina is a self-cleaning organ. Douching can actually disrupt its natural balance and lead to infection.

103

JAN	FEB	MAR	APR	MAY	JUN	JUL	AUG	SEP	OCT	NOV	DEC
1	2	3	4	5	6	7	8	9	10	11	12	13	14	15	16
17	18	19	20	21	22	23	24	25	26	27	28	29	30	31

TRACK

Phase:

Mood:

Sleep:

Energy:

Symptoms:

Temperature:

PRIORITIZE

☐

☐

☐

NOURISH

B

L

D

+

MOVE

REPLENISH

HYDRATE

💧 💧 💧 💧 💧 💧 💧 💧

"There is no limit to what we, as women, can accomplish."

—MICHELLE OBAMA

JAN	FEB	MAR	APR	MAY	JUN	JUL	AUG	SEP	OCT	NOV	DEC
1	2	3	4	5	6	7	8	9	10	11	12	13	14	15	16
17	18	19	20	21	22	23	24	25	26	27	28	29	30	31

TRACK

Phase:

Mood:

Sleep:

Energy:

Symptoms:

Temperature:

PRIORITIZE

☐

☐

☐

NOURISH

B

L

D

+

MOVE

REPLENISH

HYDRATE

💧 💧 💧 💧 💧 💧 💧 💧

TIP

Use the added creativity, motivation, and focus of the follicular phase to set goals and make a plan of attack to achieve them.

105

JAN	FEB	MAR	APR	MAY	JUN	JUL	AUG	SEP	OCT	NOV	DEC
1	2	3	4	5	6	7	8	9	10	11	12	13	14	15	16
17	18	19	20	21	22	23	24	25	26	27	28	29	30	31

TRACK

Phase:

Mood:

Sleep:

Energy:

Symptoms:

Temperature:

PRIORITIZE

- [ ]
- [ ]
- [ ]

NOURISH

B

L

D

+

MOVE

REPLENISH

HYDRATE

💧 💧 💧 💧 💧 💧 💧 💧

"Even if it has not been your habit throughout your life so far, I recommend that you learn to think positively about your body."

—INA MAY GASKIN

JAN	FEB	MAR	APR	MAY	JUN	JUL	AUG	SEP	OCT	NOV	DEC
1	2	3	4	5	6	7	8	9	10	11	12	13	14	15	16
17	18	19	20	21	22	23	24	25	26	27	28	29	30	31

TRACK

Phase:

Mood:

Sleep:

Energy:

Symptoms:

Temperature:

PRIORITIZE

☐

☐

☐

NOURISH

B

L

D

+

MOVE

REPLENISH

HYDRATE

💧 💧 💧 💧 💧 💧 💧 💧

TIP

You'll feel your sexiest during ovulation, which makes it a great time to learn about and appreciate your unique body.

JAN	FEB	MAR	APR	MAY	JUN	JUL	AUG	SEP	OCT	NOV	DEC
1	2	3	4	5	6	7	8	9	10	11	12	13	14	15	16
17	18	19	20	21	22	23	24	25	26	27	28	29	30	31

TRACK

Phase:

Mood:

Sleep:

Energy:

Symptoms:

Temperature:

PRIORITIZE

- [ ]
- [ ]
- [ ]

NOURISH

B

L

D

+

MOVE

REPLENISH

HYDRATE

💧 💧 💧 💧 💧 💧 💧 💧

"What would happen, for instance, if suddenly, magically, men could menstruate and women could not? The answer is clear—menstruation would become an enviable, boast-worthy, masculine event."

—GLORIA STEINEM

108

JAN	FEB	MAR	APR	MAY	JUN	JUL	AUG	SEP	OCT	NOV	DEC
1	2	3	4	5	6	7	8	9	10	11	12	13	14	15	16
17	18	19	20	21	22	23	24	25	26	27	28	29	30	31

TRACK

Phase:

Mood:

Sleep:

Energy:

Symptoms:

Temperature:

PRIORITIZE

☐
☐
☐

NOURISH

B

L

D

+

MOVE

REPLENISH

HYDRATE

TIP

Many wellness systems are built on circadian rhythm (the body's natural twenty-four-hour cycle) and not the menstrual cycle, which is an infradian rhythm (cycles that span weeks or months). Cycle syncing takes both into account.

JAN	FEB	MAR	APR	MAY	JUN	JUL	AUG	SEP	OCT	NOV	DEC
1	2	3	4	5	6	7	8	9	10	11	12	13	14	15	16
17	18	19	20	21	22	23	24	25	26	27	28	29	30	31

TRACK

Phase:

Mood:

Sleep:

Energy:

Symptoms:

Temperature:

PRIORITIZE

- [ ]
- [ ]
- [ ]

NOURISH

B

L

D

+

MOVE

REPLENISH

HYDRATE

💧 💧 💧 💧 💧 💧 💧 💧

"A woman is like a tea bag—you never know how strong she is until she gets in hot water."

—ELEANOR ROOSEVELT

JAN	FEB	MAR	APR	MAY	JUN	JUL	AUG	SEP	OCT	NOV	DEC
1	2	3	4	5	6	7	8	9	10	11	12	13	14	15	16
17	18	19	20	21	22	23	24	25	26	27	28	29	30	31

TRACK

Phase:

Mood:

Sleep:

Energy:

Symptoms:

Temperature:

PRIORITIZE

☐

☐

☐

NOURISH

B

L

D

+

MOVE

REPLENISH

HYDRATE

💧 💧 💧 💧 💧 💧 💧 💧

TIP

Herbal tea is great for balancing hormones during the luteal phase. Ginger, peppermint, and raspberry teas are particularly helpful (and tasty).

111

JAN	FEB	MAR	APR	MAY	JUN	JUL	AUG	SEP	OCT	NOV	DEC
1	2	3	4	5	6	7	8	9	10	11	12	13	14	15	16
17	18	19	20	21	22	23	24	25	26	27	28	29	30	31

TRACK

Phase:

Mood:

Sleep:

Energy:

Symptoms:

Temperature:

PRIORITIZE

- [ ]
- [ ]
- [ ]

NOURISH

B

L

D

+

MOVE

REPLENISH

HYDRATE

"At the end of the day, your health is your responsibility."

—JILLIAN MICHAELS

JAN	FEB	MAR	APR	MAY	JUN	JUL	AUG	SEP	OCT	NOV	DEC
1	2	3	4	5	6	7	8	9	10	11	12	13	14	15	16
17	18	19	20	21	22	23	24	25	26	27	28	29	30	31

TRACK

Phase:

Mood:

Sleep:

Energy:

Symptoms:

Temperature:

PRIORITIZE

- [ ]
- [ ]
- [ ]

NOURISH

B

L

D

+

MOVE

REPLENISH

HYDRATE

TIP

During menstruation, add more vitamin C (like citrus, berries, and bell peppers) to your diet to help you absorb more iron.

JAN	FEB	MAR	APR	MAY	JUN	JUL	AUG	SEP	OCT	NOV	DEC
1	2	3	4	5	6	7	8	9	10	11	12	13	14	15	16
17	18	19	20	21	22	23	24	25	26	27	28	29	30	31

TRACK

Phase:

Mood:

Sleep:

Energy:

Symptoms:

Temperature:

PRIORITIZE

- [ ]
- [ ]
- [ ]

NOURISH

B

L

D

+

MOVE

REPLENISH

HYDRATE

💧 💧 💧 💧 💧 💧 💧

"Above all, be the heroine of your life, not the victim."

—NORA EPHRON

JAN	FEB	MAR	APR	MAY	JUN	JUL	AUG	SEP	OCT	NOV	DEC
1	2	3	4	5	6	7	8	9	10	11	12
13	14	15	16	17	18	19	20	21	22	23	24
25	26	27	28	29	30	31					

TRACK

Phase:

Mood:

Sleep:

Energy:

Symptoms:

Temperature:

PRIORITIZE

☐

☐

☐

NOURISH

B

L

D

+

MOVE

REPLENISH

HYDRATE

💧 💧 💧 💧 💧 💧 💧

TIP

Endocrine disruptors can mess with your hormone levels, particularly in the follicular phase. Avoiding plastic dishware, food with pesticides, and products that contain heavy chemicals can help.

115

JAN	FEB	MAR	APR	MAY	JUN	JUL	AUG	SEP	OCT	NOV	DEC
1	2	3	4	5	6	7	8	9	10	11	12	13	14	15	16
17	18	19	20	21	22	23	24	25	26	27	28	29	30	31

TRACK

Phase:

Mood:

Sleep:

Energy:

Symptoms:

Temperature:

PRIORITIZE

- [ ]
- [ ]
- [ ]

NOURISH

B

L

D

+

MOVE

REPLENISH

HYDRATE

💧 💧 💧 💧 💧 💧 💧 💧

"Beauty begins the moment you decide to be yourself."

—COCO CHANEL

JAN	FEB	MAR	APR	MAY	JUN	JUL	AUG	SEP	OCT	NOV	DEC
1	2	3	4	5	6	7	8	9	10	11	12	13	14	15	16
17	18	19	20	21	22	23	24	25	26	27	28	29	30	31

TRACK

Phase:

Mood:

Sleep:

Energy:

Symptoms:

Temperature:

MOVE

REPLENISH

PRIORITIZE

☐

☐

☐

NOURISH

B

L

D

+

HYDRATE

💧 💧 💧 💧 💧 💧 💧 💧

TIP

Ovulation gives you a natural glow and flush, which means you can leave your blush in your makeup bag for a few days.

117

JAN	FEB	MAR	APR	MAY	JUN	JUL	AUG	SEP	OCT	NOV	DEC
1	2	3	4	5	6	7	8	9	10	11	12	13	14	15	16
17	18	19	20	21	22	23	24	25	26	27	28	29	30	31

TRACK

Phase:

Mood:

Sleep:

Energy:

Symptoms:

Temperature:

PRIORITIZE

- [ ]
- [ ]
- [ ]

NOURISH

B

L

D

+

MOVE

REPLENISH

HYDRATE

💧 💧 💧 💧 💧 💧 💧 💧

"When we give ourselves compassion, we are opening our hearts in a way that can transform our lives."

—DR. KRISTIN NEFF

JAN	FEB	MAR	APR	MAY	JUN	JUL	AUG	SEP	OCT	NOV	DEC
1	2	3	4	5	6	7	8	9	10	11	12	13	14	15	16
17	18	19	20	21	22	23	24	25	26	27	28	29	30	31

TRACK

Phase:

Mood:

Sleep:

Energy:

Symptoms:

Temperature:

PRIORITIZE

- [ ]
- [ ]
- [ ]

NOURISH

B

L

D

+

MOVE

REPLENISH

HYDRATE

TIP

Self-criticism can peak during the luteal phase. Breathe through it and remind yourself that you're doing your best.

JAN	FEB	MAR	APR	MAY	JUN	JUL	AUG	SEP	OCT	NOV	DEC
1	2	3	4	5	6	7	8	9	10	11	12	13	14	15	16
17	18	19	20	21	22	23	24	25	26	27	28	29	30	31

TRACK

Phase:

Mood:

Sleep:

Energy:

Symptoms:

Temperature:

PRIORITIZE

- [ ]
- [ ]
- [ ]

NOURISH

B

L

D

+

MOVE

REPLENISH

HYDRATE

"Alone we can do so little. Together we can do so much."

—HELEN KELLER

JAN	FEB	MAR	APR	MAY	JUN	JUL	AUG	SEP	OCT	NOV	DEC
1	2	3	4	5	6	7	8	9	10	11	12	13	14	15	16
17	18	19	20	21	22	23	24	25	26	27	28	29	30	31

TRACK

Phase:

Mood:

Sleep:

Energy:

Symptoms:

Temperature:

PRIORITIZE

- [ ]
- [ ]
- [ ]

NOURISH

B

L

D

+

MOVE

REPLENISH

HYDRATE

TIP

Surround yourself with good people. Studies show that women who feel supported during their periods have an easier time dealing with symptoms.

121

JAN	FEB	MAR	APR	MAY	JUN	JUL	AUG	SEP	OCT	NOV	DEC
1	2	3	4	5	6	7	8	9	10	11	12	13	14	15	16
17	18	19	20	21	22	23	24	25	26	27	28	29	30	31

TRACK

Phase:

Mood:

Sleep:

Energy:

Symptoms:

Temperature:

PRIORITIZE

☐

☐

☐

NOURISH

B

L

D

+

MOVE

REPLENISH

HYDRATE

💧 💧 💧 💧 💧 💧 💧 💧

"The most alluring thing a woman can have is confidence."

—BEYONCÉ

JAN	FEB	MAR	APR	MAY	JUN	JUL	AUG	SEP	OCT	NOV	DEC
1	2	3	4	5	6	7	8	9	10	11	12	13	14	15	16
17	18	19	20	21	22	23	24	25	26	27	28	29	30	31

TRACK

Phase:

Mood:

Sleep:

Energy:

Symptoms:

Temperature:

PRIORITIZE

☐
☐
☐

NOURISH

B

L

D

+

MOVE

REPLENISH

HYDRATE

💧 💧 💧 💧 💧 💧 💧 💧

TIP

Increased estrogen during the follicular phase will make your hair look thicker and healthier. Take advantage of it and update those headshots!

JAN	FEB	MAR	APR	MAY	JUN	JUL	AUG	SEP	OCT	NOV	DEC
1	2	3	4	5	6	7	8	9	10	11	12	13	14	15	16
17	18	19	20	21	22	23	24	25	26	27	28	29	30	31

TRACK

Phase:

Mood:

Sleep:

Energy:

Symptoms:

Temperature:

PRIORITIZE

- [ ]
- [ ]
- [ ]

NOURISH

B

L

D

+

MOVE

REPLENISH

HYDRATE

💧 💧 💧 💧 💧 💧 💧 💧

"I don't think I'll ever grow old and say, 'What was I thinking eating all those fruits and vegetables?'"

—NANCY S. MURE

JAN	FEB	MAR	APR	MAY	JUN	JUL	AUG	SEP	OCT	NOV	DEC
1	2	3	4	5	6	7	8	9	10	11	12	13	14	15	16
17	18	19	20	21	22	23	24	25	26	27	28	29	30	31

TRACK

Phase:

Mood:

Sleep:

Energy:

Symptoms:

Temperature:

PRIORITIZE

- [ ]
- [ ]
- [ ]

NOURISH

B

L

D

+

MOVE

REPLENISH

HYDRATE

TIP

Eating healthy, whole foods is a major part of cycle syncing because nutrients derived from food are more effective and easily absorbed than nutrients derived from supplements.

125

JAN	FEB	MAR	APR	MAY	JUN	JUL	AUG	SEP	OCT	NOV	DEC
1	2	3	4	5	6	7	8	9	10	11	12	13	14	15	16
17	18	19	20	21	22	23	24	25	26	27	28	29	30	31

TRACK

Phase:

Mood:

Sleep:

Energy:

Symptoms:

Temperature:

PRIORITIZE

☐

☐

☐

NOURISH

B

L

D

+

MOVE

REPLENISH

HYDRATE

💧 💧 💧 💧 💧 💧 💧 💧

"The body knows things beyond the mind's understanding. Trust its wisdom and follow its lead."

—CAROLINE MYSS

JAN	FEB	MAR	APR	MAY	JUN	JUL	AUG	SEP	OCT	NOV	DEC
1	2	3	4	5	6	7	8	9	10	11	12	13	14	15	16
17	18	19	20	21	22	23	24	25	26	27	28	29	30	31

TRACK

Phase:

Mood:

Sleep:

Energy:

Symptoms:

Temperature:

PRIORITIZE

- [ ]
- [ ]
- [ ]

NOURISH

B

L

D

+

MOVE

REPLENISH

HYDRATE

TIP

If you experience breast tenderness during the luteal phase, try cutting back on caffeine and alcohol, which can exacerbate the issue.

127

JAN	FEB	MAR	APR	MAY	JUN	JUL	AUG	SEP	OCT	NOV	DEC
1	2	3	4	5	6	7	8	9	10	11	12	13	14	15	16
17	18	19	20	21	22	23	24	25	26	27	28	29	30	31

TRACK

Phase:

Mood:

Sleep:

Energy:

Symptoms:

Temperature:

PRIORITIZE

☐

☐

☐

NOURISH

B

L

D

+

MOVE

REPLENISH

HYDRATE

💧 💧 💧 💧 💧 💧 💧 💧

"Self-care is not selfish. You cannot serve from an empty vessel."

—ELEANOR BROWN

JAN	FEB	MAR	APR	MAY	JUN	JUL	AUG	SEP	OCT	NOV	DEC
1	2	3	4	5	6	7	8	9	10	11	12	13	14	15	16
17	18	19	20	21	22	23	24	25	26	27	28	29	30	31

TRACK

Phase:

Mood:

Sleep:

Energy:

Symptoms:

Temperature:

PRIORITIZE

☐

☐

☐

NOURISH

B

L

D

+

MOVE

REPLENISH

HYDRATE

💧 💧 💧 💧 💧 💧 💧

TIP

If you find exercising helps with your menstrual cramps, but you don't have much energy, try yoga, Pilates, or other lower-impact workouts.

JAN	FEB	MAR	APR	MAY	JUN	JUL	AUG	SEP	OCT	NOV	DEC
1	2	3	4	5	6	7	8	9	10	11	12	13	14	15	16
17	18	19	20	21	22	23	24	25	26	27	28	29	30	31

TRACK

Phase:

Mood:

Sleep:

Energy:

Symptoms:

Temperature:

PRIORITIZE

☐

☐

☐

NOURISH

B

L

D

+

MOVE

REPLENISH

HYDRATE

💧 💧 💧 💧 💧 💧 💧 💧

"Learn to embrace your own unique beauty; celebrate your unique gifts . . . imperfections are actually a gift."

—KERRY WASHINGTON

JAN	FEB	MAR	APR	MAY	JUN	JUL	AUG	SEP	OCT	NOV	DEC
1	2	3	4	5	6	7	8	9	10	11	12	13	14	15	16
17	18	19	20	21	22	23	24	25	26	27	28	29	30	31

TRACK

Phase:

Mood:

Sleep:

Energy:

Symptoms:

Temperature:

PRIORITIZE

- [ ]
- [ ]
- [ ]

NOURISH

B

L

D

+

MOVE

REPLENISH

HYDRATE

TIP

When the follicular phase imbues you with added confidence, put it to good use. Do something fun or inspiring that you've been hesitant to do.

JAN	FEB	MAR	APR	MAY	JUN	JUL	AUG	SEP	OCT	NOV	DEC
1	2	3	4	5	6	7	8	9	10	11	12	13	14	15	16
17	18	19	20	21	22	23	24	25	26	27	28	29	30	31

TRACK

Phase:

Mood:

Sleep:

Energy:

Symptoms:

Temperature:

PRIORITIZE

☐

☐

☐

NOURISH

B

L

D

+

MOVE

REPLENISH

HYDRATE

💧 💧 💧 💧 💧 💧 💧 💧

"I am learning to trust the journey even when I do not understand it."

—MILA BRON

132

JAN	FEB	MAR	APR	MAY	JUN	JUL	AUG	SEP	OCT	NOV	DEC
1	2	3	4	5	6	7	8	9	10	11	12	13	14	15	16
17	18	19	20	21	22	23	24	25	26	27	28	29	30	31

TRACK

Phase:

Mood:

Sleep:

Energy:

Symptoms:

Temperature:

PRIORITIZE

- [ ]
- [ ]
- [ ]

NOURISH

B

L

D

+

MOVE

REPLENISH

HYDRATE

TIP

Your cervix can change positions and soften during the ovulatory phase, so you may find that you enjoy certain sexual positions even more.

JAN	FEB	MAR	APR	MAY	JUN	JUL	AUG	SEP	OCT	NOV	DEC
1	2	3	4	5	6	7	8	9	10	11	12	13	14	15	16
17	18	19	20	21	22	23	24	25	26	27	28	29	30	31

TRACK

Phase:

Mood:

Sleep:

Energy:

Symptoms:

Temperature:

PRIORITIZE

☐

☐

☐

NOURISH

B

L

D

+

MOVE

REPLENISH

HYDRATE

💧 💧 💧 💧 💧 💧 💧 💧

"Self-care is how you take your power back."

—LALAH DELIA

JAN	FEB	MAR	APR	MAY	JUN	JUL	AUG	SEP	OCT	NOV	DEC
1	2	3	4	5	6	7	8	9	10	11	12	13	14	15	16
17	18	19	20	21	22	23	24	25	26	27	28	29	30	31

TRACK

Phase:

Mood:

Sleep:

Energy:

Symptoms:

Temperature:

PRIORITIZE

☐

☐

☐

NOURISH

B

L

D

+

MOVE

REPLENISH

HYDRATE

💧 💧 💧 💧 💧 💧 💧

TIP

Tracking your cycle keeps you accountable to yourself. Seeing your routine in print helps you prioritize caring for your body and mind.

JAN	FEB	MAR	APR	MAY	JUN	JUL	AUG	SEP	OCT	NOV	DEC
1	2	3	4	5	6	7	8	9	10	11	12	13	14	15	16
17	18	19	20	21	22	23	24	25	26	27	28	29	30	31

TRACK

Phase:

Mood:

Sleep:

Energy:

Symptoms:

Temperature:

PRIORITIZE

- [ ]
- [ ]
- [ ]

NOURISH

B

L

D

+

MOVE

REPLENISH

HYDRATE

💧 💧 💧 💧 💧 💧 💧

"Remain calm, because peace equals power."
—JOYCE MEYER

JAN	FEB	MAR	APR	MAY	JUN	JUL	AUG	SEP	OCT	NOV	DEC
1	2	3	4	5	6	7	8	9	10	11	12	13	14	15	16
17	18	19	20	21	22	23	24	25	26	27	28	29	30	31

TRACK

Phase:

Mood:

Sleep:

Energy:

Symptoms:

Temperature:

PRIORITIZE

- [ ]
- [ ]
- [ ]

NOURISH

B

L

D

+

MOVE

REPLENISH

HYDRATE

TIP

When you're craving a sweet treat in the luteal phase, opt for antioxidant-rich dark chocolate, which can boost your mood and promote feelings of well-being.

JAN	FEB	MAR	APR	MAY	JUN	JUL	AUG	SEP	OCT	NOV	DEC
1	2	3	4	5	6	7	8	9	10	11	12	13	14	15	16
17	18	19	20	21	22	23	24	25	26	27	28	29	30	31

TRACK

Phase:

Mood:

Sleep:

Energy:

Symptoms:

Temperature:

PRIORITIZE

- [ ]
- [ ]
- [ ]

NOURISH

B

L

D

+

MOVE

REPLENISH

HYDRATE

💧 💧 💧 💧 💧 💧 💧 💧

"Sometimes courage is the quiet voice at the end of the day saying, 'I will try again tomorrow.'"

—MARY ANNE RADMACHER

JAN	FEB	MAR	APR	MAY	JUN	JUL	AUG	SEP	OCT	NOV	DEC
1	2	3	4	5	6	7	8	9	10	11	12	13	14	15	16
17	18	19	20	21	22	23	24	25	26	27	28	29	30	31

TRACK

Phase:

Mood:

Sleep:

Energy:

Symptoms:

Temperature:

PRIORITIZE

- [ ]
- [ ]
- [ ]

NOURISH

B

L

D

+

MOVE

REPLENISH

HYDRATE

TIP

Sleeping on your side or sleeping in the fetal position can combat cramps by relieving pressure on your abdominal muscles.

JAN	FEB	MAR	APR	MAY	JUN	JUL	AUG	SEP	OCT	NOV	DEC
1	2	3	4	5	6	7	8	9	10	11	12	13	14	15	16
17	18	19	20	21	22	23	24	25	26	27	28	29	30	31	

TRACK

Phase:

Mood:

Sleep:

Energy:

Symptoms:

Temperature:

PRIORITIZE

☐

☐

☐

NOURISH

B

L

D

+

MOVE

REPLENISH

HYDRATE

💧 💧 💧 💧 💧 💧 💧 💧

"Each day comes bearing its gifts.
Untie the ribbon."

—ANN RUTH SCHABACKER

140

JAN	FEB	MAR	APR	MAY	JUN	JUL	AUG	SEP	OCT	NOV	DEC
1	2	3	4	5	6	7	8	9	10	11	12	13	14	15	16
17	18	19	20	21	22	23	24	25	26	27	28	29	30	31

TRACK

Phase:

Mood:

Sleep:

Energy:

Symptoms:

Temperature:

PRIORITIZE

☐

☐

☐

NOURISH

B

L

D

+

MOVE

REPLENISH

HYDRATE

💧 💧 💧 💧 💧 💧 💧

TIP

The follicular phase is a great time to try new foods. It can heighten your senses, making you more likely to catch subtle scents or flavors.

141

JAN	FEB	MAR	APR	MAY	JUN	JUL	AUG	SEP	OCT	NOV	DEC
1	2	3	4	5	6	7	8	9	10	11	12	13	14	15	16
17	18	19	20	21	22	23	24	25	26	27	28	29	30	31

TRACK

Phase:

Mood:

Sleep:

Energy:

Symptoms:

Temperature:

PRIORITIZE

- [ ]
- [ ]
- [ ]

NOURISH

B

L

D

+

MOVE

REPLENISH

HYDRATE

○ ○ ○ ○ ○ ○ ○ ○

"Be strong, be fearless, be beautiful."

—MISTY COPELAND

JAN	FEB	MAR	APR	MAY	JUN	JUL	AUG	SEP	OCT	NOV	DEC
1	2	3	4	5	6	7	8	9	10	11	12	13	14	15	16
17	18	19	20	21	22	23	24	25	26	27	28	29	30	31

TRACK

Phase:

Mood:

Sleep:

Energy:

Symptoms:

Temperature:

PRIORITIZE

☐

☐

☐

NOURISH

B

L

D

+

MOVE

REPLENISH

HYDRATE

💧 💧 💧 💧 💧 💧 💧 💧

TIP

Your voice may get higher when you're ovulating because of an unconscious biological desire to sound more feminine, giving you an edge at karaoke night.

143

JAN	FEB	MAR	APR	MAY	JUN	JUL	AUG	SEP	OCT	NOV	DEC
1	2	3	4	5	6	7	8	9	10	11	12	13	14	15	16
17	18	19	20	21	22	23	24	25	26	27	28	29	30	31

TRACK

Phase:

Mood:

Sleep:

Energy:

Symptoms:

Temperature:

PRIORITIZE

- [ ]
- [ ]
- [ ]

NOURISH

B

L

D

+

MOVE

REPLENISH

HYDRATE

💧 💧 💧 💧 💧 💧 💧 💧

"Nature has given us all the pieces required to achieve exceptional wellness and health but has left it to us to put these pieces together."

—DIANE McLAREN

JAN	FEB	MAR	APR	MAY	JUN	JUL	AUG	SEP	OCT	NOV	DEC
1	2	3	4	5	6	7	8	9	10	11	12	13	14	15	16
17	18	19	20	21	22	23	24	25	26	27	28	29	30	31

TRACK

Phase:

Mood:

Sleep:

Energy:

Symptoms:

Temperature:

PRIORITIZE

- [ ]
- [ ]
- [ ]

NOURISH

B

L

D

+

MOVE

REPLENISH

HYDRATE

TIP

Soak up some sunshine and breathe in the fresh air. Connecting with nature can help you regulate your emotions during your luteal phase.

JAN	FEB	MAR	APR	MAY	JUN	JUL	AUG	SEP	OCT	NOV	DEC
1	2	3	4	5	6	7	8	9	10	11	12	13	14	15	16
17	18	19	20	21	22	23	24	25	26	27	28	29	30	31

TRACK

Phase:

Mood:

Sleep:

Energy:

Symptoms:

Temperature:

PRIORITIZE

- [ ]
- [ ]
- [ ]

NOURISH

B

L

D

+

MOVE

REPLENISH

HYDRATE

💧 💧 💧 💧 💧 💧 💧 💧

"The most difficult thing is the decision to act; the rest is merely tenacity."

—AMELIA EARHART

JAN	FEB	MAR	APR	MAY	JUN	JUL	AUG	SEP	OCT	NOV	DEC
1	2	3	4	5	6	7	8	9	10	11	12	13	14	15	16
17	18	19	20	21	22	23	24	25	26	27	28	29	30	31

TRACK

Phase:

Mood:

Sleep:

Energy:

Symptoms:

Temperature:

PRIORITIZE

- [ ]
- [ ]
- [ ]

NOURISH

B

L

D

+

MOVE

REPLENISH

HYDRATE

TIP

If cramps are keeping you from seizing the day, you may find some relief in taking supplements like magnesium, a B-vitamin complex, and fish oil.

JAN	FEB	MAR	APR	MAY	JUN	JUL	AUG	SEP	OCT	NOV	DEC
1	2	3	4	5	6	7	8	9	10	11	12	13	14	15	16
17	18	19	20	21	22	23	24	25	26	27	28	29	30	31

TRACK

Phase:

Mood:

Sleep:

Energy:

Symptoms:

Temperature:

PRIORITIZE

- [ ]
- [ ]
- [ ]

NOURISH

B

L

D

+

MOVE

REPLENISH

HYDRATE

💧 💧 💧 💧 💧 💧 💧 💧

"When life is sweet, say thank you and celebrate. And when life is bitter, say thank you and grow."

—SHAUNA NIEQUIST

148

JAN	FEB	MAR	APR	MAY	JUN	JUL	AUG	SEP	OCT	NOV	DEC
1	2	3	4	5	6	7	8	9	10	11	12	13	14	15	16
17	18	19	20	21	22	23	24	25	26	27	28	29	30	31

TRACK

Phase:

Mood:

Sleep:

Energy:

Symptoms:

Temperature:

PRIORITIZE

- [ ]
- [ ]
- [ ]

NOURISH

B

L

D

+

MOVE

REPLENISH

HYDRATE

💧 💧 💧 💧 💧 💧 💧 💧

TIP

Having a shorter follicular phase can make it more difficult to conceive, but it's not a definitive factor. Tracking your cycle can help you have more productive conversations with your healthcare provider.

JAN	FEB	MAR	APR	MAY	JUN	JUL	AUG	SEP	OCT	NOV	DEC
1	2	3	4	5	6	7	8	9	10	11	12	13	14	15	16
17	18	19	20	21	22	23	24	25	26	27	28	29	30	31

TRACK

Phase:

Mood:

Sleep:

Energy:

Symptoms:

Temperature:

PRIORITIZE

☐

☐

☐

NOURISH

B

L

D

+

MOVE

REPLENISH

HYDRATE

💧 💧 💧 💧 💧 💧 💧

"So much of what happens in life is out of your control, but how you respond to it is in your control."

—HILLARY RODHAM CLINTON

JAN	FEB	MAR	APR	MAY	JUN	JUL	AUG	SEP	OCT	NOV	DEC
1	2	3	4	5	6	7	8	9	10	11	12	13	14	15	16
17	18	19	20	21	22	23	24	25	26	27	28	29	30	31

TRACK

Phase:

Mood:

Sleep:

Energy:

Symptoms:

Temperature:

PRIORITIZE

☐
☐
☐

NOURISH

B

L

D

+

MOVE

REPLENISH

HYDRATE

TIP

Tailoring your exercise routine to the phases of your cycle and how you're feeling each day can keep you from overworking your body and help you balance your hormones and cortisol levels naturally.

JAN	FEB	MAR	APR	MAY	JUN	JUL	AUG	SEP	OCT	NOV	DEC
1	2	3	4	5	6	7	8	9	10	11	12	13	14	15	16
17	18	19	20	21	22	23	24	25	26	27	28	29	30	31

TRACK

Phase:

Mood:

Sleep:

Energy:

Symptoms:

Temperature:

MOVE

REPLENISH

PRIORITIZE

- [ ]
- [ ]
- [ ]

NOURISH

B

L

D

+

HYDRATE

💧 💧 💧 💧 💧 💧 💧 💧

"When in doubt, choose change."
—LILY LEUNG

JAN	FEB	MAR	APR	MAY	JUN	JUL	AUG	SEP	OCT	NOV	DEC
1	2	3	4	5	6	7	8	9	10	11	12	13	14	15	16
17	18	19	20	21	22	23	24	25	26	27	28	29	30	31

TRACK

Phase:

Mood:

Sleep:

Energy:

Symptoms:

Temperature:

PRIORITIZE

- ☐
- ☐
- ☐

NOURISH

B

L

D

+

MOVE

REPLENISH

HYDRATE

💧 💧 💧 💧 💧 💧 💧 💧

TIP

Feeling bloated during the luteal phase? Avoid drinking carbonated beverages, chewing gum, and using a straw to enjoy your beverages (noncarbonated and otherwise).

JAN	FEB	MAR	APR	MAY	JUN	JUL	AUG	SEP	OCT	NOV	DEC
1	2	3	4	5	6	7	8	9	10	11	12
13	14	15	16	17	18	19	20	21	22	23	24
25	26	27	28	29	30	31					

TRACK

Phase:

Mood:

Sleep:

Energy:

Symptoms:

Temperature:

PRIORITIZE

☐

☐

☐

NOURISH

B

L

D

+

MOVE

REPLENISH

HYDRATE

💧 💧 💧 💧 💧 💧 💧 💧

"When you can't find your purpose in a day, make it to look after yourself."

—DODIE CLARK

JAN	FEB	MAR	APR	MAY	JUN	JUL	AUG	SEP	OCT	NOV	DEC
1	2	3	4	5	6	7	8	9	10	11	12	13	14	15	16
17	18	19	20	21	22	23	24	25	26	27	28	29	30	31

TRACK

Phase:

Mood:

Sleep:

Energy:

Symptoms:

Temperature:

PRIORITIZE

☐

☐

☐

NOURISH

B

L

D

+

MOVE

REPLENISH

HYDRATE

💧 💧 💧 💧 💧 💧 💧

TIP

Brain fog getting to you during your period? Exercise—especially a walk in the sunshine—can help.

JAN	FEB	MAR	APR	MAY	JUN	JUL	AUG	SEP	OCT	NOV	DEC
1	2	3	4	5	6	7	8	9	10	11	12	13	14	15	16
17	18	19	20	21	22	23	24	25	26	27	28	29	30	31

TRACK

Phase:

Mood:

Sleep:

Energy:

Symptoms:

Temperature:

PRIORITIZE

- [ ]
- [ ]
- [ ]

NOURISH

B

L

D

+

MOVE

REPLENISH

HYDRATE

💧 💧 💧 💧 💧 💧 💧 💧

"The better you know yourself, the better your relationship with the rest of the world."

—TONI COLLETTE

JAN	FEB	MAR	APR	MAY	JUN	JUL	AUG	SEP	OCT	NOV	DEC
1	2	3	4	5	6	7	8	9	10	11	12
13	14	15	16	17	18	19	20	21	22	23	24
25	26	27	28	29	30	31					

TRACK

Phase:

Mood:

Sleep:

Energy:

Symptoms:

Temperature:

PRIORITIZE

- [ ]
- [ ]
- [ ]

NOURISH

B

L

D

+

MOVE

REPLENISH

HYDRATE

◇ ◇ ◇ ◇ ◇ ◇ ◇

TIP

Not sure whether you're in the follicular phase? Check your basal body temperature, which will be at its lowest (between 97.0°F and 97.5°F).

JAN	FEB	MAR	APR	MAY	JUN	JUL	AUG	SEP	OCT	NOV	DEC
1	2	3	4	5	6	7	8	9	10	11	12	13	14	15	16
17	18	19	20	21	22	23	24	25	26	27	28	29	30	31

TRACK

Phase:

Mood:

Sleep:

Energy:

Symptoms:

Temperature:

PRIORITIZE

☐

☐

☐

NOURISH

B

L

D

+

MOVE

REPLENISH

HYDRATE

💧 💧 💧 💧 💧 💧 💧 💧

"Growth and comfort do not coexist."

—GINNI ROMETTY

158

JAN	FEB	MAR	APR	MAY	JUN	JUL	AUG	SEP	OCT	NOV	DEC
1	2	3	4	5	6	7	8	9	10	11	12
13	14	15	16	17	18	19	20	21	22	23	24
25	26	27	28	29	30	31					

TRACK

Phase:

Mood:

Sleep:

Energy:

Symptoms:

Temperature:

MOVE

REPLENISH

PRIORITIZE

- [ ]
- [ ]
- [ ]

NOURISH

B

L

D

+

HYDRATE

💧 💧 💧 💧 💧 💧 💧 💧

TIP

Although ovulation can make you feel amazing, it can also occasionally cause headaches and nausea. Over-the-counter headache meds, hydration, and rest should have you feeling like new again.

JAN	FEB	MAR	APR	MAY	JUN	JUL	AUG	SEP	OCT	NOV	DEC
1	2	3	4	5	6	7	8	9	10	11	12	13	14	15	16
17	18	19	20	21	22	23	24	25	26	27	28	29	30	31

TRACK

Phase:

Mood:

Sleep:

Energy:

Symptoms:

Temperature:

PRIORITIZE

- [ ]
- [ ]
- [ ]

NOURISH

B

L

D

+

MOVE

REPLENISH

HYDRATE

💧 💧 💧 💧 💧 💧 💧 💧

"A year from now, you will wish you had started today."

—KAREN LAMB

JAN	FEB	MAR	APR	MAY	JUN	JUL	AUG	SEP	OCT	NOV	DEC
1	2	3	4	5	6	7	8	9	10	11	12	13	14	15	16
17	18	19	20	21	22	23	24	25	26	27	28	29	30	31

TRACK

Phase:

Mood:

Sleep:

Energy:

Symptoms:

Temperature:

PRIORITIZE

- [ ]
- [ ]
- [ ]

NOURISH

B

L

D

+

MOVE

REPLENISH

HYDRATE

💧 💧 💧 💧 💧 💧 💧

TIP

You don't have to go all-in on cycle syncing right away. Start tracking your cycle and incorporating the advice bit by bit, gradually building it into a habit.

JAN	FEB	MAR	APR	MAY	JUN	JUL	AUG	SEP	OCT	NOV	DEC
1	2	3	4	5	6	7	8	9	10	11	12	13	14	15	16
17	18	19	20	21	22	23	24	25	26	27	28	29	30	31

TRACK

Phase:

Mood:

Sleep:

Energy:

Symptoms:

Temperature:

PRIORITIZE

☐

☐

☐

NOURISH

B

L

D

+

MOVE

REPLENISH

HYDRATE

💧 💧 💧 💧 💧 💧 💧 💧

"It's hard work that makes things happen."

—SHONDA RHIMES

JAN	FEB	MAR	APR	MAY	JUN	JUL	AUG	SEP	OCT	NOV	DEC
1	2	3	4	5	6	7	8	9	10	11	12	13	14	15	16
17	18	19	20	21	22	23	24	25	26	27	28	29	30	31

TRACK

Phase:

Mood:

Sleep:

Energy:

Symptoms:

Temperature:

PRIORITIZE

☐

☐

☐

NOURISH

B

L

D

+

MOVE

REPLENISH

HYDRATE

💧 💧 💧 💧 💧 💧 💧 💧

TIP

The luteal phase sees you at your most focused and detail oriented, making it the prime time for task completion.

JAN	FEB	MAR	APR	MAY	JUN	JUL	AUG	SEP	OCT	NOV	DEC
1	2	3	4	5	6	7	8	9	10	11	12	13	14	15	16
17	18	19	20	21	22	23	24	25	26	27	28	29	30	31

TRACK

Phase:

Mood:

Sleep:

Energy:

Symptoms:

Temperature:

PRIORITIZE

☐

☐

☐

NOURISH

B

L

D

+

MOVE

REPLENISH

HYDRATE

💧 💧 💧 💧 💧 💧 💧 💧

"To know how much there is to know is the beginning of learning to live."

—DOROTHY WEST

JAN	FEB	MAR	APR	MAY	JUN	JUL	AUG	SEP	OCT	NOV	DEC
1	2	3	4	5	6	7	8	9	10	11	12	13	14	15	16
17	18	19	20	21	22	23	24	25	26	27	28	29	30	31

TRACK

Phase:

Mood:

Sleep:

Energy:

Symptoms:

Temperature:

PRIORITIZE

- [ ]
- [ ]
- [ ]

NOURISH

B

L

D

+

MOVE

REPLENISH

HYDRATE

💧 💧 💧 💧 💧 💧 💧

TIP

Period running late? It could be stress. Consider whether you've been especially tense and need to relieve some of the pressure.

JAN	FEB	MAR	APR	MAY	JUN	JUL	AUG	SEP	OCT	NOV	DEC
1	2	3	4	5	6	7	8	9	10	11	12	13	14	15	16
17	18	19	20	21	22	23	24	25	26	27	28	29	30	31

TRACK

Phase:

Mood:

Sleep:

Energy:

Symptoms:

Temperature:

PRIORITIZE

- [ ]
- [ ]
- [ ]

NOURISH

B

L

D

+

MOVE

REPLENISH

HYDRATE

💧 💧 💧 💧 💧 💧 💧

"Sometimes, you need to give yourself a break when you've had a lot of life change."

—BARBARA FREETHY

JAN	FEB	MAR	APR	MAY	JUN	JUL	AUG	SEP	OCT	NOV	DEC
1	2	3	4	5	6	7	8	9	10	11	12	13	14	15	16
17	18	19	20	21	22	23	24	25	26	27	28	29	30	31

TRACK

Phase:

Mood:

Sleep:

Energy:

Symptoms:

Temperature:

PRIORITIZE

☐

☐

☐

NOURISH

B

L

D

+

MOVE

REPLENISH

HYDRATE

TIP

Take it easy on caffeine consumption during your follicular phase, when your energy levels are naturally higher, to avoid anxiety and insomnia.

JAN	FEB	MAR	APR	MAY	JUN	JUL	AUG	SEP	OCT	NOV	DEC
1	2	3	4	5	6	7	8	9	10	11	12	13	14	15	16
17	18	19	20	21	22	23	24	25	26	27	28	29	30	31

TRACK

Phase:

Mood:

Sleep:

Energy:

Symptoms:

Temperature:

PRIORITIZE

- [ ]
- [ ]
- [ ]

NOURISH

B

L

D

+

MOVE

REPLENISH

HYDRATE

💧 💧 💧 💧 💧 💧 💧 💧

"Take care of yourself, be healthy, and always believe you can be successful in anything you truly want."

—ALESSANDRA AMBROSIO

JAN	FEB	MAR	APR	MAY	JUN	JUL	AUG	SEP	OCT	NOV	DEC
1	2	3	4	5	6	7	8	9	10	11	12	13	14	15	16
17	18	19	20	21	22	23	24	25	26	27	28	29	30	31

TRACK

Phase:

Mood:

Sleep:

Energy:

Symptoms:

Temperature:

PRIORITIZE

- [ ]
- [ ]
- [ ]

NOURISH

B

L

D

+

MOVE

REPLENISH

HYDRATE

△ △ △ △ △ △ △ △

TIP

Cycle syncing's benefits to your mental and physical well-being reach far beyond your monthly cycle. A life rich in exercise, self-care, and nourishing foods is good for your heart, brain, bones, and immune system.

JAN	FEB	MAR	APR	MAY	JUN	JUL	AUG	SEP	OCT	NOV	DEC
1	2	3	4	5	6	7	8	9	10	11	12	13	14	15	16
17	18	19	20	21	22	23	24	25	26	27	28	29	30	31

TRACK

Phase:

Mood:

Sleep:

Energy:

Symptoms:

Temperature:

PRIORITIZE

☐

☐

☐

NOURISH

B

L

D

+

MOVE

REPLENISH

HYDRATE

💧 💧 💧 💧 💧 💧 💧 💧

"Take the time today to love yourself. You deserve it."

—AVINA CELESTE

JAN	FEB	MAR	APR	MAY	JUN	JUL	AUG	SEP	OCT	NOV	DEC
1	2	3	4	5	6	7	8	9	10	11	12	13	14	15	16
17	18	19	20	21	22	23	24	25	26	27	28	29	30	31

TRACK

Phase:

Mood:

Sleep:

Energy:

Symptoms:

Temperature:

PRIORITIZE

- [ ]
- [ ]
- [ ]

NOURISH

B

L

D

+

MOVE

REPLENISH

HYDRATE

TIP

You deserve to feel good in your body. Do something today that makes you feel that way, whether it's taking a nap, getting some exercise, or enjoying a warm cup of tea.

JAN	FEB	MAR	APR	MAY	JUN	JUL	AUG	SEP	OCT	NOV	DEC
1	2	3	4	5	6	7	8	9	10	11	12	13	14	15	16
17	18	19	20	21	22	23	24	25	26	27	28	29	30	31

TRACK

Phase:

Mood:

Sleep:

Energy:

Symptoms:

Temperature:

PRIORITIZE

- [ ]
- [ ]
- [ ]

NOURISH

B

L

D

+

MOVE

REPLENISH

HYDRATE

💧 💧 💧 💧 💧 💧 💧 💧

"Your health is what you make of it. Everything you do and think either adds to the vitality, energy, and spirit you possess or takes away from it."

—ANN WIGMORE

JAN	FEB	MAR	APR	MAY	JUN	JUL	AUG	SEP	OCT	NOV	DEC
1	2	3	4	5	6	7	8	9	10	11	12	13	14	15	16
17	18	19	20	21	22	23	24	25	26	27	28	29	30	31

TRACK

Phase:

Mood:

Sleep:

Energy:

Symptoms:

Temperature:

PRIORITIZE

- [ ]
- [ ]
- [ ]

NOURISH

B

L

D

+

MOVE

REPLENISH

HYDRATE

💧 💧 💧 💧 💧 💧 💧

TIP

A particularly heavy or painful period can be your body's way of alerting you to an underlying issue, such as endometriosis. Make sure you talk to your healthcare provider.

JAN	FEB	MAR	APR	MAY	JUN	JUL	AUG	SEP	OCT	NOV	DEC
1	2	3	4	5	6	7	8	9	10	11	12	13	14	15	16
17	18	19	20	21	22	23	24	25	26	27	28	29	30	31

TRACK

Phase:

Mood:

Sleep:

Energy:

Symptoms:

Temperature:

PRIORITIZE

- [ ]
- [ ]
- [ ]

NOURISH

B

L

D

+

MOVE

REPLENISH

HYDRATE

💧 💧 💧 💧 💧 💧 💧 💧

"A strong woman understands that gifts such as logic, decisiveness, and strength are just as feminine as intuition and emotional connection."

—NANCY RATHBURN

JAN	FEB	MAR	APR	MAY	JUN	JUL	AUG	SEP	OCT	NOV	DEC
1	2	3	4	5	6	7	8	9	10	11	12	13	14	15	16
17	18	19	20	21	22	23	24	25	26	27	28	29	30	31

TRACK

Phase:

Mood:

Sleep:

Energy:

Symptoms:

Temperature:

PRIORITIZE

☐

☐

☐

NOURISH

B

L

D

+

MOVE

REPLENISH

HYDRATE

💧 💧 💧 💧 💧 💧 💧 💧

TIP

Higher levels of estradiol during the follicular phase help you feel happier and more focused—an ideal combination when you need to make tough decisions.

175

JAN	FEB	MAR	APR	MAY	JUN	JUL	AUG	SEP	OCT	NOV	DEC
1	2	3	4	5	6	7	8	9	10	11	12	13	14	15	16
17	18	19	20	21	22	23	24	25	26	27	28	29	30	31

TRACK

Phase:

Mood:

Sleep:

Energy:

Symptoms:

Temperature:

PRIORITIZE

☐

☐

☐

NOURISH

B

L

D

+

MOVE

REPLENISH

HYDRATE

💧 💧 💧 💧 💧 💧 💧 💧

"If you obey all the rules, you miss all the fun."

—KATHARINE HEPBURN

176

JAN	FEB	MAR	APR	MAY	JUN	JUL	AUG	SEP	OCT	NOV	DEC
1	2	3	4	5	6	7	8	9	10	11	12	13	14	15	16
17	18	19	20	21	22	23	24	25	26	27	28	29	30	31

TRACK

Phase:

Mood:

Sleep:

Energy:

Symptoms:

Temperature:

PRIORITIZE

☐

☐

☐

NOURISH

B

L

D

+

MOVE

REPLENISH

HYDRATE

💧 💧 💧 💧 💧 💧 💧

TIP

A higher libido and more open mind during the ovulatory phase make it the perfect time to try something new in bed.

JAN	FEB	MAR	APR	MAY	JUN	JUL	AUG	SEP	OCT	NOV	DEC
1	2	3	4	5	6	7	8	9	10	11	12	13	14	15	16
17	18	19	20	21	22	23	24	25	26	27	28	29	30	31

TRACK

Phase:

Mood:

Sleep:

Energy:

Symptoms:

Temperature:

PRIORITIZE

- [ ]
- [ ]
- [ ]

NOURISH

B

L

D

+

MOVE

REPLENISH

HYDRATE

💧 💧 💧 💧 💧 💧 💧 💧

"Just because you make a good plan, doesn't mean that's what's gonna happen."

—TAYLOR SWIFT

JAN	FEB	MAR	APR	MAY	JUN	JUL	AUG	SEP	OCT	NOV	DEC
1	2	3	4	5	6	7	8	9	10	11	12	13	14	15	16
17	18	19	20	21	22	23	24	25	26	27	28	29	30	31

TRACK

Phase:

Mood:

Sleep:

Energy:

Symptoms:

Temperature:

PRIORITIZE

- [ ]
- [ ]
- [ ]

NOURISH

B

L

D

+

MOVE

REPLENISH

HYDRATE

💧 💧 💧 💧 💧 💧 💧 💧

TIP

If you've been tracking your cycle and implementing these tips, and you're still experiencing uncomfortable symptoms, talk to your healthcare provider. An underlying issue may be to blame.

JAN	FEB	MAR	APR	MAY	JUN	JUL	AUG	SEP	OCT	NOV	DEC
1	2	3	4	5	6	7	8	9	10	11	12	13	14	15	16
17	18	19	20	21	22	23	24	25	26	27	28	29	30	31

TRACK

Phase:

Mood:

Sleep:

Energy:

Symptoms:

Temperature:

PRIORITIZE

☐

☐

☐

NOURISH

B

L

D

+

MOVE

REPLENISH

HYDRATE

💧 💧 💧 💧 💧 💧 💧 💧

"If you don't like the road you're walking, start paving another one."

—DOLLY PARTON

JAN	FEB	MAR	APR	MAY	JUN	JUL	AUG	SEP	OCT	NOV	DEC
1	2	3	4	5	6	7	8	9	10	11	12	13	14	15	16
17	18	19	20	21	22	23	24	25	26	27	28	29	30	31

TRACK

Phase:

Mood:

Sleep:

Energy:

Symptoms:

Temperature:

PRIORITIZE

- [ ]
- [ ]
- [ ]

NOURISH

B

L

D

+

MOVE

REPLENISH

HYDRATE

TIP

The luteal phase's clarity and assertiveness make it the perfect time to cut out what's not working in your life and decide on a new way forward.

JAN	FEB	MAR	APR	MAY	JUN	JUL	AUG	SEP	OCT	NOV	DEC
1	2	3	4	5	6	7	8	9	10	11	12	13	14	15	16
17	18	19	20	21	22	23	24	25	26	27	28	29	30	31

TRACK

Phase:

Mood:

Sleep:

Energy:

Symptoms:

Temperature:

PRIORITIZE

☐

☐

☐

NOURISH

B

L

D

+

MOVE

REPLENISH

HYDRATE

💧 💧 💧 💧 💧 💧 💧 💧

"No woman can call herself free who does not own and control her body."

—MARGARET SANGER

JAN	FEB	MAR	APR	MAY	JUN	JUL	AUG	SEP	OCT	NOV	DEC
1	2	3	4	5	6	7	8	9	10	11	12	13	14	15	16
17	18	19	20	21	22	23	24	25	26	27	28	29	30	31

TRACK

Phase:

Mood:

Sleep:

Energy:

Symptoms:

Temperature:

PRIORITIZE

- [ ]
- [ ]
- [ ]

NOURISH

B

L

D

+

MOVE

REPLENISH

HYDRATE

TIP

It's still possible to get pregnant during your period, so make sure you're using protection if pregnancy isn't your goal.

JAN	FEB	MAR	APR	MAY	JUN	JUL	AUG	SEP	OCT	NOV	DEC
1	2	3	4	5	6	7	8	9	10	11	12	13	14	15	16
17	18	19	20	21	22	23	24	25	26	27	28	29	30	31

TRACK

Phase:

Mood:

Sleep:

Energy:

Symptoms:

Temperature:

PRIORITIZE

- [ ]
- [ ]
- [ ]

NOURISH

B

L

D

+

MOVE

REPLENISH

HYDRATE

💧 💧 💧 💧 💧 💧 💧 💧

"A woman's health is her capital."
—HARRIET BEECHER STOWE

JAN	FEB	MAR	APR	MAY	JUN	JUL	AUG	SEP	OCT	NOV	DEC
1	2	3	4	5	6	7	8	9	10	11	12	13	14	15	16
17	18	19	20	21	22	23	24	25	26	27	28	29	30	31

TRACK

Phase:

Mood:

Sleep:

Energy:

Symptoms:

Temperature:

PRIORITIZE

- [ ]
- [ ]
- [ ]

NOURISH

B

L

D

+

MOVE

REPLENISH

HYDRATE

TIP

Some naturopaths believe that the phytoestrogens in flax seeds and the zinc in pumpkin seeds can help balance your hormones during the follicular phase.

JAN	FEB	MAR	APR	MAY	JUN	JUL	AUG	SEP	OCT	NOV	DEC
1	2	3	4	5	6	7	8	9	10	11	12	13	14	15	16
17	18	19	20	21	22	23	24	25	26	27	28	29	30	31

TRACK

Phase:

Mood:

Sleep:

Energy:

Symptoms:

Temperature:

PRIORITIZE

☐

☐

☐

NOURISH

B

L

D

+

MOVE

REPLENISH

HYDRATE

💧 💧 💧 💧 💧 💧 💧 💧

"Today is your day to start fresh, to eat right, to train hard, to live healthy, to be proud."

—BONNIE PFIESTER

JAN	FEB	MAR	APR	MAY	JUN	JUL	AUG	SEP	OCT	NOV	DEC
1	2	3	4	5	6	7	8	9	10	11	12	13	14	15	16
17	18	19	20	21	22	23	24	25	26	27	28	29	30	31

TRACK

Phase:

Mood:

Sleep:

Energy:

Symptoms:

Temperature:

PRIORITIZE

☐
☐
☐

NOURISH

B

L

D

+

MOVE

REPLENISH

HYDRATE

TIP

Have you gotten off-track with your cycle syncing? Start again. Even if you miss a few days (or weeks), you can still accumulate enough information over time to help you hone your habits and feel your best.

JAN	FEB	MAR	APR	MAY	JUN	JUL	AUG	SEP	OCT	NOV	DEC
1	2	3	4	5	6	7	8	9	10	11	12	13	14	15	16
17	18	19	20	21	22	23	24	25	26	27	28	29	30	31

TRACK

Phase:

Mood:

Sleep:

Energy:

Symptoms:

Temperature:

PRIORITIZE

- [ ]
- [ ]
- [ ]

NOURISH

B

L

D

+

MOVE

REPLENISH

HYDRATE

💧 💧 💧 💧 💧 💧 💧 💧

"There is purpose in your season of waiting."

—MEGAN SMALLEY

JAN	FEB	MAR	APR	MAY	JUN	JUL	AUG	SEP	OCT	NOV	DEC
1	2	3	4	5	6	7	8	9	10	11	12	13	14	15	16
17	18	19	20	21	22	23	24	25	26	27	28	29	30	31

TRACK

Phase:

Mood:

Sleep:

Energy:

Symptoms:

Temperature:

PRIORITIZE

- [ ]
- [ ]
- [ ]

NOURISH

B

L

D

+

MOVE

REPLENISH

HYDRATE

💧 💧 💧 💧 💧 💧 💧 💧

TIP

The autumn of your cycle (your luteal phase) helps clear the way for the rest of your cycle, which makes it a great time for looking inward and reflecting.

JAN	FEB	MAR	APR	MAY	JUN	JUL	AUG	SEP	OCT	NOV	DEC
1	2	3	4	5	6	7	8	9	10	11	12	13	14	15	16
17	18	19	20	21	22	23	24	25	26	27	28	29	30	31

TRACK

Phase:

Mood:

Sleep:

Energy:

Symptoms:

Temperature:

PRIORITIZE

☐

☐

☐

NOURISH

B

L

D

+

MOVE

REPLENISH

HYDRATE

💧 💧 💧 💧 💧 💧 💧 💧

"You celebrate what works and take tender care of what doesn't, with lotion, polish, and kindness."

—ANNE LAMOTT

JAN	FEB	MAR	APR	MAY	JUN	JUL	AUG	SEP	OCT	NOV	DEC
1	2	3	4	5	6	7	8	9	10	11	12	13	14	15	16
17	18	19	20	21	22	23	24	25	26	27	28	29	30	31

TRACK

Phase:

Mood:

Sleep:

Energy:

Symptoms:

Temperature:

PRIORITIZE

☐

☐

☐

NOURISH

B

L

D

+

MOVE

REPLENISH

HYDRATE

💧 💧 💧 💧 💧 💧 💧 💧

TIP

Exercise can relieve period symptoms, but rest can be just as beneficial. This is your permission slip to skip your workout.

JAN	FEB	MAR	APR	MAY	JUN	JUL	AUG	SEP	OCT	NOV	DEC
1	2	3	4	5	6	7	8	9	10	11	12	13	14	15	16
17	18	19	20	21	22	23	24	25	26	27	28	29	30	31

TRACK

Phase:

Mood:

Sleep:

Energy:

Symptoms:

Temperature:

PRIORITIZE

☐

☐

☐

NOURISH

B

L

D

+

MOVE

REPLENISH

HYDRATE

💧 💧 💧 💧 💧 💧 💧 💧

*"You do not find the happy life.
You make it."*

—CAMILLA EYRING KIMBALL

JAN	FEB	MAR	APR	MAY	JUN	JUL	AUG	SEP	OCT	NOV	DEC
1	2	3	4	5	6	7	8	9	10	11	12	13	14	15	16
17	18	19	20	21	22	23	24	25	26	27	28	29	30	31

TRACK

Phase:

Mood:

Sleep:

Energy:

Symptoms:

Temperature:

PRIORITIZE

- ☐
- ☐
- ☐

NOURISH

B

L

D

+

MOVE

REPLENISH

HYDRATE

💧 💧 💧 💧 💧 💧 💧 💧

TIP

Keep the refined carbs (e.g., bread, pastries, and beer) to a minimum to avoid consistently elevating your insulin, as high insulin could prevent you from ovulating regularly.

JAN	FEB	MAR	APR	MAY	JUN	JUL	AUG	SEP	OCT	NOV	DEC
1	2	3	4	5	6	7	8	9	10	11	12	13	14	15	16
17	18	19	20	21	22	23	24	25	26	27	28	29	30	31

TRACK

Phase:

Mood:

Sleep:

Energy:

Symptoms:

Temperature:

PRIORITIZE

☐

☐

☐

NOURISH

B

L

D

+

MOVE

REPLENISH

HYDRATE

💧 💧 💧 💧 💧 💧 💧 💧

"You may have to fight a battle more than once to win it."

—MARGARET THATCHER

194

JAN	FEB	MAR	APR	MAY	JUN	JUL	AUG	SEP	OCT	NOV	DEC
1	2	3	4	5	6	7	8	9	10	11	12	13	14	15	16
17	18	19	20	21	22	23	24	25	26	27	28	29	30	31

TRACK

Phase:

Mood:

Sleep:

Energy:

Symptoms:

Temperature:

PRIORITIZE

☐

☐

☐

NOURISH

B

L

D

+

MOVE

REPLENISH

HYDRATE

💧 💧 💧 💧 💧 💧 💧 💧

TIP

Cycle syncing takes time and tweaking. What worked last month may not work this month. Have patience. This journey isn't about doing everything perfectly. It's about doing and feeling your best.

JAN	FEB	MAR	APR	MAY	JUN	JUL	AUG	SEP	OCT	NOV	DEC
1	2	3	4	5	6	7	8	9	10	11	12	13	14	15	16
17	18	19	20	21	22	23	24	25	26	27	28	29	30	31

TRACK

Phase:

Mood:

Sleep:

Energy:

Symptoms:

Temperature:

PRIORITIZE

- [ ]
- [ ]
- [ ]

NOURISH

B

L

D

+

MOVE

REPLENISH

HYDRATE

"The challenge is not to be perfect . . . it's to be whole."

—JANE FONDA

JAN	FEB	MAR	APR	MAY	JUN	JUL	AUG	SEP	OCT	NOV	DEC
1	2	3	4	5	6	7	8	9	10	11	12	13	14	15	16
17	18	19	20	21	22	23	24	25	26	27	28	29	30	31

TRACK

Phase:

Mood:

Sleep:

Energy:

Symptoms:

Temperature:

PRIORITIZE

- [ ]
- [ ]
- [ ]

NOURISH

B

L

D

+

MOVE

REPLENISH

HYDRATE

💧 💧 💧 💧 💧 💧 💧

TIP

Some pain during your cycle may be "normal," but that doesn't mean you should suffer through it. Talk to your healthcare provider about ways to feel your best.

197

MONTH:

Activity Planner

SUNDAY	MONDAY	TUESDAY	WEDNESDAY

THURSDAY	FRIDAY	SATURDAY

NOTES

MONTH:

Activity Planner

SUNDAY	MONDAY	TUESDAY	WEDNESDAY

THURSDAY	FRIDAY	SATURDAY

NOTES

MONTH:

Activity Planner

SUNDAY	MONDAY	TUESDAY	WEDNESDAY

THURSDAY	FRIDAY	SATURDAY

NOTES

MONTH:

Activity Planner

SUNDAY	MONDAY	TUESDAY	WEDNESDAY

THURSDAY	FRIDAY	SATURDAY

NOTES

MONTH:

Activity Planner

SUNDAY	MONDAY	TUESDAY	WEDNESDAY

THURSDAY	FRIDAY	SATURDAY

NOTES

MONTH:

Activity Planner

SUNDAY	MONDAY	TUESDAY	WEDNESDAY

THURSDAY	FRIDAY	SATURDAY

NOTES

MONTH:

Activity Planner

SUNDAY	MONDAY	TUESDAY	WEDNESDAY

THURSDAY	FRIDAY	SATURDAY

NOTES

MONTH:

Activity Planner

SUNDAY	MONDAY	TUESDAY	WEDNESDAY

THURSDAY	FRIDAY	SATURDAY

NOTES

MONTH:

Activity Planner

SUNDAY	MONDAY	TUESDAY	WEDNESDAY

THURSDAY	FRIDAY	SATURDAY

NOTES

MONTH:

Activity Planner

SUNDAY	MONDAY	TUESDAY	WEDNESDAY

THURSDAY	FRIDAY	SATURDAY

NOTES

MONTH:

Activity Planner

SUNDAY	MONDAY	TUESDAY	WEDNESDAY

THURSDAY	FRIDAY	SATURDAY

NOTES

MONTH:

Activity Planner

SUNDAY	MONDAY	TUESDAY	WEDNESDAY

THURSDAY	FRIDAY	SATURDAY

NOTES

Cycle Tracker

Use the tracker on the opposite page to get a big-picture overview of your cycle. You'll learn how long yours is (which you can input below) and be able to see patterns in your symptoms that can inform your routines. You might use colors to indicate your bleeding days and symbols for your symptoms. This is your private guide to your cycle, so make it your own.

TRACKER KEY	
Light Bleeding	
Heavy Bleeding	
Spotting	
Missed Period	
Ovulating	
Cramps	
Cravings	
Acne	
Headache	
Migraine	
Tired	
Angry	
Sad	
Energized	
Strong	
Happy	

CYCLE LENGTH	
January	
February	
March	
April	
May	
June	
July	
August	
September	
October	
November	
December	

	J	F	M	A	M	J	J	A	S	O	N	D
1												
2												
3												
4												
5												
6												
7												
8												
9												
10												
11												
12												
13												
14												
15												
16												
17												
18												
19												
20												
21												
22												
23												
24												
25												
26												
27												
28												
29												
30												
31												

	J	F	M	A	M	J	J	A	S	O	N	D
1												
2												
3												
4												
5												
6												
7												
8												
9												
10												
11												
12												
13												
14												
15												
16												
17												
18												
19												
20												
21												
22												
23												
24												
25												
26												
27												
28												
29												
30												
31												